T0251666

OSCEs for the MRCOG Part 2

OSCEs for the MRCOG Part 2: A Self-Assessment Guide

2nd edition

Tony Hollingworth
Consultant in Obstetrics & Gynaecology, Whipps Cross University
Hospital Trust, London, UK

Janice Rymer
Professor of Obstetrics & Gynaecology, Dean of Undergraduate
Medicine, Guy's & St Thomas' Foundation Hospital Trust,
King's College, London, UK

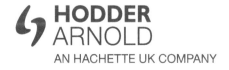
HODDER
ARNOLD
AN HACHETTE UK COMPANY

First published in Great Britain in 2005 by Hodder Education
This second edition published in 2011 by
Hodder Arnold, an imprint of Hodder Education, a division of Hachette UK

338 Euston Road, London NW1 3BH

http://www.hodderarnold.com

British Library Cataloguing in Publication Data
A catalogue record for this book is available from the British Library

Library of Congress Cataloging-in-Publication Data
A catalog record for this book is available from the Library of Congress

ISBN 978 1 4441 2184 1

1 2 3 4 5 6 7 8 9 10

Commissioning Editors:	Gavin Jamieson/Francesca Naish
Project Editors:	Sarah Penny/Mischa Barrett
Production Controller:	Joanna Walker
Cover Design:	Amina Dudhia

Typeset in Palatino Light 10.5 pt by Phoenix Photosetting, Chatham, Kent
Printed and bound in India by Replika Press

What do you think about this book? Or any other Hodder Arnold title?
Please visit our website: www.hodderarnold.com

DEDICATION

This book is dedicated to our support systems: Ann, Roger, Victoria, Chloe and Adam.

CONTENTS

Foreword to first edition   ix

Preface   x

Acknowledgements   xi

List of abbreviations used   xii

Introduction   xiv

REVIEW STATIONS

1. Gynaecology history   1
2. Early pregnancy problem-management   9
3. Prioritization on delivery suite   13
4. Surgical skills – placenta praevia   19
5. Communication skills – ectopic mismanagement   23
6. Premenstrual syndrome   27
7. Breaking bad news – anencephaly   33
8. Infertility – case notes   39
9. Audit   48
10. Obstetric history   52

CIRCUIT A

1. Breaking bad news   59
2. Preoperative ward round   65
3. Obstetric history and management   69
4. Management problem – gynaecology   73
5. Prenatal counselling   77
6. Obstetric emergency – uterine inversion   81
7. Operating list prioritization   84
8. Bereavement   89
9. Emergency contraception   93
10. Intermenstrual bleeding   97

CIRCUIT B

1. Labour ward prioritization   100
2. Abdominal pain – premature labour   107

3. Urinary incontinence   111
4. Prioritization of GP letters   117
5. Operative – Caesarean section   131
6. Abnormal smear   135
7. CTG abnormality   139
8. Interactive viva   145
9. Ectopic pregnancy – explain laparoscopy   153
10. Breech delivery   157

CIRCUIT C

1. Medical ethics and the law – preparatory station   161
2. Shoulder dystocia – teaching station   167
3. Ovarian cyst   171
4. Intraoperative complication – debriefing a patient   177
5. Postpartum haemorrhage – structured viva   181
6. Obstetric history with travel   185
7. Secondary amenorrhoea – structured viva   191
8. Twin pregnancy – structured viva   195
9. Molar pregnancy – counselling with result   201
10. Results interpretation – preparatory station   205

CIRCUIT D

1. Breaking bad news – Down's syndrome   215
2. Pregnancy case – structured viva   219
3. Antepartum haemorrhage – structured viva   223
4. Clinical governance – preparatory station   229
5. Fertility issues   235
6. Management of ectopic pregnancy – structured viva   241
7. Secondary amenorrhoea – role-play   245
8. Postoperative pelvic abscess – role-play   249
9. Polycystic ovary syndrome – structured viva   253
10. Audit – preparatory station   257

Index   261

FOREWORD TO FIRST EDITION

Achieving success in the MRCOG marks the beginning of joining a profession in which there must be continued professional development and learning. It is a hurdle to be conquered. Knowledge is not enough, technique is important.

The authors, Antony Hollingworth and Janice Rymer, are respected and experienced examiners used to setting marking schemes for the OSCE. This work will be an invaluable aid to study and self assessment. The scenarios used are all comparable to those met in the exam, and the properly prepared candidate would be well advised to consider using this book.

Roger Baldwin

PREFACE

The examination for membership for the Royal College of Obstetricians and Gynaecologists aims to set a standard of competent, safe practice for anyone pursuing a career in obstetrics and gynaecology. The oral part of the examination now consists of Objective Structured Clinical Examinations (OSCEs). We have both been past chairs of the RCOG OSCE Committee, and convenors of the RCOG Part 2 course. We therefore have extensive experience in teaching and preparing candidates for this examination, and in examining candidates. In this new edition we have tried to update the questions and give comprehensive examples of the type of OSCEs that may appear in the exam. Advice is given on how to approach these stations and the common problems that we have seen candidates encounter.

Since the first edition of this book, clinical governance has become an increasingly important aspect of how we deliver care. Questions on clinical governance are therefore included in this book as there is every likelihood that this aspect of practice may feature somewhere in the MRCOG exam.

Remember that the written part of the examination concentrates on your knowledge, and the OSCEs will assess your application of knowledge, and skills. In our specialty, communication skills are especially important and we would hope that by going through this book and practising the OSCEs stations you will be competent in all the skills that the Royal College of Obstetricians and Gynaecologists expects you to have. We hope that you find this book invaluable in your preparation for the examination and we wish you luck.

Tony Hollingworth and Janice Rymer

ACKNOWLEDGEMENTS

We would like to thank all the people who bought the first edition of our book and hopefully gained some insight into the OSCE part of the MRCOG exam and became members of the RCOG.

In updating this book, we would like to thank the team at Hodder who have helped bring this second edition to fruition and also kept us on track, namely Gavin, Francesca, Sarah, Mischa and Joanna. We would also like to thank our proofreader, Vivienne.

Once again we would like to acknowledge Roger Baldwin, who wrote the foreword to the first edition. He has significantly influenced not only our approach to learning and teaching but also that of numerous others who attended the Whipps Cross MRCOG course over the many years that he ran it.

Tony Hollingworth and Janice Rymer

LIST OF ABBREVIATIONS USED

A&E	Accident and Emergency
AF	atrial fibrillation
AFP	alpha-fetoprotein
APH	ante partum haemorrhage
ARM	artificial rupture of membranes
BMI	body mass index
BP	blood pressure
BSO	bilateral salpingo-ophorectomy
CDH	congenital dislocation of the hip
CF	cystic fibrosis
CRP	C-reactive protein
CS	Caesarean section
CTG	cardiotocograph
CVP	central venous pressure
CVS	chorionic villus sampling
D&C	dilation and curettage
DIC	disseminated intravascular coagulation
DUB	dysfunctional uterine bleeding
DVT	deep vein thrombosis
ECV	external cephalic version
EDC	expected date of confinement
EDD	expected date of delivery
ERPC	evacuation of retained products of conception
EUA	examination under anaesthetic
FBC	full blood count
FBS	fetal blood sampling
FFP	fresh frozen plasma
FSH	follicle-stimulating hormone
GA	general anaesthetic
GDM	gestational diabetes mellitus
GnRH	gonadotrophin-releasing hormone
GP	general practitioner
GTT	glucose tolerance test
Hb	haemoglobin
HCG	human chorionic gonadotropin
HRT	hormone replacement therapy
HSG	hysterosalpingogram
HVS	high vaginal swab
ICSI	intracytoplasmic sperm injection
ICU	intensive care unit
IDDM	insulin-dependent diabetes mellitus
IMB	intermenstrual bleeding
IUFD	intrauterine fetal demise
IUGR	intrauterine growth restriction
IUI	intrauterine insemination
IUP	intrauterine pressure

IUS	intrauterine system
IVF	in-vitro fertilization
JW	Jehovah's Witness
LFT	liver function test
LH	luteinizing hormone
LLETZ	large loop excision of the transformation zone
LMP	last menstrual period
LSCS	lower-segment Caesarean section
MCV	mean corpuscular volume
MDT	multidisciplinary team
MRSA	methicillin-resistant *Staph. aureus*
MSU	mid-stream urine
NG	nasogastric
NTD	neural tube defect
O&G	obstetrics and gynaecology
OCP	oral contraceptive pill
ODA	operating department assistant
OP	occiput posterior (position)
OT	occiput transverse (position)
PALS	Patient Advice and Liaison Service
PCC	postcoital contraception
PCOS	polycystic ovary syndrome
PE	pulmonary embolism
PET	pre-eclamptic toxaemia
PID	pelvic inflammatory disease
PMB	postmenopausal bleeding
PMS	premenstrual syndrome
POD	Pouch of Douglas
POP	progesterone-only pill
PPH	postpartum haemorrhage
PPROM	premature prelabour rupture of membranes
RMI	relative malignant index
RSL	right sacro-lateral
SHBG	sex-hormone-binding globulin
SHO	senior house officer
SpR	specialist registrar
SRM	spontaneous rupture of membranes
SSRI	selective serotonin reuptake inhibitor
ST1	specialty trainee year 1
STD	sexually transmitted disease
SVD	spontaneous vaginal delivery
TAH	total abdominal hysterectomy
TED	thromboembolic deterrent
TOP	termination of pregnancy
U&E	urea and electrolytes
USS	ultrasound scan
UTI	urinary tract infection
VBAC	vaginal birth after Caesarean section
VDRL	Venereal Disease research laboratory
VE	vaginal examination
VTE	venous thromboembolism
WBC	white blood cell count
WCC	white cell count

INTRODUCTION

In the MRCOG Part 2 examination, knowledge is tested in the written paper by multiple-choice questions (30 per cent), extended matching questions (40 per cent) and short essays (30 per cent). Clinical skills are tested in an objective structured clinical examination (OSCE) which replaces the traditional clinical long case and viva voce. The OSCE is designed to produce a valid and reproducible assessment of your skills. The MRCOG is a licensing examination and therefore the examination is not norm-referenced but criterion-referenced. This means that the minimum standard acceptable is decided before the test and you either reach that standard and pass, or you go below it and fail. This is much fairer than a norm-referenced examination where you may be disadvantaged if you go through with an experienced cohort of students or, likewise, you may be advantaged if you go through with a less experienced cohort.

The two parts are stand-alone exams and you have to pass both parts in order to be awarded the MRCOG. Each diet of exam is 'blueprinted' so that the exam as a whole covers the entire curriculum. No two diets are exactly the same and that is the reason why you have to pass both parts in the same diet of exams. In short, if you pass the written and fail the OSCE then you have to sit the whole exam again.

In the OSCE, each candidate is exposed to the same set of scenarios. This means that the examination is reproducible and the marking is standardized. As you are exposed to ten different examiners, this improves the reliability of the examination.

The MRCOG Part 2 OSCE is a series of examinations based on clinical skills applied in a range of contexts where there is wide sampling with a structured assessment, and this improves the reliability.

About the examination

The OSCE currently consists of ten marked stations and two preparatory stations. Each station lasts 15 minutes, and the total duration of the examination is 3 hours. One minute before the conclusion of the station (at 14 minutes) there will be a bell to conclude your involvement and to allow the examiner to mark it. When this bell goes, the candidate should move to the next station and read the relevant information. All the information relating to the station will be posted outside it as well as on the desk within the station. Take as much time as you need to read the information. You need to ensure you have read the question thoroughly; once you have grasped it, proceed into the station. This may take a few minutes but you are in control of your time. Do not be rushed. If you have just had a difficult station, you may need an extra minute or two to recover. As the information will be outside the station, this means that you will be in control of your timing. If you need the time, take it and make sure that you are calm and composed before you enter the next station.

This is a professional examination and respect for patients (role-players) is important. You should dress appropriately and be well groomed. You should be polite, friendly and transmit an air of confidence and competence to both the role-players and the examiners.

At the stations where there are role-players, introduce yourself by your full name (first name only is too casual) and do your normal greeting. This may involve a handshake. Speak slowly and clearly and make eye-contact. The role-players may have been instructed to behave in a certain way – so be mindful of their body language and attitude.

Of the 10 stations where an examiner is present, the candidate has to perform a task and each task tests certain skills, communication or problem-solving abilities. Depending on the type of station there may be a role-player, some form of imaging, a pelvic model, surgical instruments or a clinical scenario. As the examination evolves, new types of station will be brought in. Currently the examination may include the following areas.

History-taking

This is a core skill and is usually included at every exam. Each candidate should be able to score very highly, but surprisingly the marks for this type of test are consistently low. It is important to take a comprehensive history, not only of the presenting complaint but of all the relevant past histories. One logical approach is to ask an open-ended question about the patient's presentation and then comprehensively go through the presenting complaint; then go to past obstetric and gynaecology history and with the previous pregnancies note whether there were any problems, whether they were induced or spontaneous labour, whether there was a normal delivery and whether there were any intrapartum and/or postpartum problems. The weight and sex of the babies should be recorded. If there are any miscarriages or terminations, it is important to know whether evacuations were performed and whether there were any postoperative problems. A functional enquiry of all the systems should be undertaken, followed by medication history (which includes alcohol, smoking and recreational drug use), known allergies, family history and social history.

Remember that the patient may have been briefed to be difficult or non-communicative.

When there is a role-player at the station, it is essential that you do not interact with the examiner who is there as an observer. If you do, this will completely break up the rapport that you have developed with the role-player. If you run out of questions and the consultation becomes silent, do not approach the examiner. In all role-playing stations the examiner will not have any information for you; all the necessary information to score marks will be on the instruction sheet. There should be no reason to question any examination findings, as the mark scheme will reflect issues around the information given. In other words, the questions are not designed to catch you out.

Good practice

- Introduce yourself.
- Remain professional.
- Stay in control of the consultation.
- Ask whether the patient has understood your questions.
- Ask whether she (or sometimes he) has any questions.
- Summarise the information back to the role player.
- Practise with a friend.
- Studying a video of yourself is very useful.

Clinical skills

With this type of station any skill that you perform in the wards, in the clinics or in the operating theatre could be tested, depending on the feasibility of setting up the station. These stations should be easy as it is what you do every day at work. You just need to transpose yourself mentally into the situation and do what you normally do. This kind of question may include demonstrating with a manikin (e.g. a forceps delivery); it could also involve you teaching a role-player to acquire certain skills.

Counselling skills

These stations will have a role-player and may involve breaking bad news or dealing with an anxious or angry patient. The role-players will have been well briefed to act in a certain way. It is essential that you avoid medical jargon. Clearly you need to be empathetic and compassionate in these situations. Always consider the appropriateness of drawing a diagram to help the role-player to understand.

Prioritization

This is about your ability to set priorities in clinical work. It may involve a busy labour ward, calls you may receive from the ward or the rest of the hospital, or operating list priorities. It is important to be familiar with waiting times, such as target referrals for suspected cancers and the 62-day rule, 18-week routine wait for surgery from time of referral.

Logical thought

This area covers the ability to design an audit, protocol, or information sheet, or critique a medical journal paper, protocol or patient information pamphlet. This may well be an article from the internet that you are asked to discuss with the examiner or the role-player.

With these stations you must have an opinion as to whether the document/information is of good or poor quality, peer-reviewed or not, any hidden agenda (e.g. money) and be able to defend your opinion. You must be able to give an overview of the documents, as well as addressing some details.

Clinical management of gynaecological or obstetric problems

Here you may be faced with a scenario in either the clinic or the operating theatre and you must describe to the examiner what your management would be. You may be given examination findings or results that you may need to interpret.

Communication stations

Any scenario that may occur in your working day can be tested here. At these stations knowledge is often secondary and it is how you interact with the role-player that is important. If the 'patient' is angry, allow her to talk but keep control of the situation. Do not take that anger personally; the role-player will have been told to act that way. If the 'patient' is upset, let her talk, and act as though you have all the time in the world.

Structured oral examination/viva

At these stations the examiner will ask set questions to which you need to provide the answers. The make-up of these stations may be very varied, from a preoperative ward round to a surgical viva. The station may be a sequential viva looking over a patient journey/course of a pregnancy and once a section has been completed you cannot go back to a previous part. We have tried to include most of the types of structured viva you will come across.

Clinical governance

This may involve audit or looking over a set of notes with a poor outcome and discussing, with either the examiner or the role-player, what was happening in her care. If something has gone wrong, what recommendations would you make for the future for her and also generically?

Role-players

The actors used for the exam are very able at improvisation. The person in front of you may not be a physical match for the one in the stated clinical scenario. However, it is important to appreciate that this aspect (e.g. raised BMI) will be taken into account in the allocation of marks. Role-players can award up to 2 marks depending on their confidence in the doctor and whether they would be prepared to see the candidate again.

Marking

The marking of all the stations is structured and thereby objective. This means that whichever examiner you get, you should score the same mark. The examiners have practised the questions, by role-playing themselves as both the candidate and the examiner. The design of the OSCE ensures that, as far as possible, each candidate is exposed to the same examination.

At the stations where there is a role-player and an examiner, do not interact with the examiner; he or she is merely an observer. To do well in the examination, all you need to do is to perform all your clinical activities as you would normally do them. Go back to what you would do in the clinic, ward, theatre or labour ward. This is a licensing examination and the RCOG needs to be sure you are competent.

REVIEW STATION 1

Gynaecology history

Candidate's instructions

The patient you are about to see has been referred to your gynaecology outpatient clinic by her GP. A copy of the referral letter is given below. Read the letter and obtain a relevant history from the patient. You should discuss any relevant investigations and treatment options with the patient.

The Surgery
Large Pond Road
London SE16

Dear Gynaecologist

Please would you see Joan Dunn, aged 45 years? She is a female solicitor who has a 2-year history of painful heavy periods. She bleeds for 10 days every month and is in so much pain she is bedridden throughout some of her period. She is fed up and wants something done.

This patient is overweight with a body mass index (BMI) of 30 kg/m^2 and on examination she has a large pelvic mass. An ultrasound scan has revealed this to be fibroids with an anterior fundal fibroid $12 \times 8 \times 6$ cm and a submucosal fibroid $3 \times 4 \times 4$ cm.

Thank you for your help.

Yours sincerely

Dr W White MRCGP

> **MARKS WILL BE AWARDED FOR YOUR ABILITY TO TAKE A HISTORY AND TO EXPLAIN THE APPROPRIATE INVESTIGATIONS AND TREATMENT PLAN TO THE PATIENT.**

Role-player's brief

- You are Joan Dunn, a 45-year-old solicitor. Your attitude should be that of a friendly and calm patient who is generally interested to find out all the benefits and risks of the treatment of your problem. You may, however, turn combative if you are treated with discourtesy or belittled, or if you are generally dissatisfied with the doctor's attitude. After all, you are a busy professional woman and do not want to be treated as though you are not very bright. You are worried that you may have cancer of the womb as your sister has that problem as well.
- Let the doctor know if you do not understand any medical terms. Let him or her lead in the discussion and do not interrupt unless you need some clarification. You may prompt the doctor (see below) at the end if he/she asks whether you have any questions.
- Your periods started when you were 13, and had been regular until recently, each period lasting about 3 days, coming every 28–30 days.
- However, over the last 8 months, you have noticed that you have experienced bleeding in between your periods and they are irregular. This occurs irregularly when you are expected to be dry. You have to wear pads every day and are generally worried. You do not have bleeding after sexual intercourse.
- You have seen a GP who gave you some iron tablets but these did not seem to stop your periods. No other medications were given to you.
- Your last cervical smear was done 3 years ago and that was normal.
- You have noticed that you have become more lethargic over the last 3 months, although you have not had any chest pain, shortness of breath or palpitations.
- You have not been pregnant before as you and your husband have been rather busy with your careers and you do not intend to get pregnant.
- You have had diabetes for the last 5 years and have been very careful with your diet. Your yearly checks with your diabetes nurse have shown that your control has been good. You do not have any other symptoms.
- You have no drug allergy.
- There is a family history of diabetes and cancer of the womb. Your mother suffers from diabetes controlled with medication. Your sister was 39 years old when she was diagnosed with early cancer of the womb. She had an operation to remove the womb and has been well since.
- You occasionally drink alcohol and do not smoke.

Prompts

1. What do I have?
2. What needs to be done for me?

Examiner's instructions and mark sheet

History

- Symptoms – details of intramenstrual bleeding (IMB) – date of last menstrual period (LMP)
- Previous menstrual history including smear history
- Previous obstetric history
- Family history (and patient anxiety)
- Social history, including smoking, alcohol, recreational drugs
- Any fertility issues

0   1   2   3   4   5   6

Investigations

- Full blood count (FBC)
- Blood glucose
- Glycosylated haemoglobin
- Cervical smear
- Pelvic ultrasound scan (ovaries and endometrial pathology)
- Pipelle biopsy of endometrium ± hysteroscopy
- Endometrial sample (re RCOG guidelines on dysfunctional bleeding)
- Assessment of possible therapeutic options, conservative and surgical

0   1   2   3   4   5   6

Further management dependent on findings

- Hysteroscopy and assessment of suitability for resection of submucosal fibroid if pipelle normal
- Hysterectomy if histology abnormal or for definitive treatment
- Low risk of malignancy (reassure patient)
- Could take cyclical hormone tablets if no specific abnormality found
- Even if nothing abnormal is found, patient encouraged to report further IMB
- Suggest ongoing active supervision of diabetes, and weight loss
- Discuss role of oophorectomy if patient decides on hysterectomy

0   1   2   3   4   5   6

Role-player's score

0   1   2

(2 = role-player happy to see candidate again, 1 = prepared to see candidate again, 0 = never wants to see candidate again).

Total: /20

Discussion

What does this station aim to test?

Taking a gynaecology history is a core skill for an MRCOG candidate. This is a skill that you practise every day and you should be very good at it. Notoriously, candidates score very badly on history-taking stations.

You are also being tested on your communication skills, so you must be sensitive to the problem but also must be very thorough in obtaining a complete history. In these stations the patients may be briefed to be difficult and may try to lead you up the wrong path. You must therefore be in control of the consultation while at the same time communicating well.

What are the pitfalls?

Many candidates are not very thorough when they take a history and, in particular, forget to enquire about family history and social history. In this day and age, one should always enquire about alcohol and illicit drug use.

At this station you have also been asked to discuss relevant investigations and treatment options with the patient. This means that you must outline the investigations, but as you are not given the results, you have to propose the treatment options depending on the results of the investigation. You must therefore be clear in your thinking as to how to get this across simply to the patient so that she can understand. It may be helpful to draw a diagram.

Your preparation

As you do this every day, it is easy to practise but you need to be supervised to ensure that you are being thorough. In the exam, marks will also be awarded for being systematic rather than gleaning the information in a random fashion. The best way to practise this station is to use a real patient and ask a colleague to observe you.

Early pregnancy problem-management

Candidate's instructions

You are working in the early pregnancy assessment unit and the patient you are about to see has just had an ultrasound scan. You have not met her before. The results of the scan are as follows:

TRANSVAGINAL SCAN

- Anteverted uterus
- Fetal pole identified in uterus
- No fetal heart activity
- Sac consistent with 5 weeks' gestation
- Both ovaries appear normal
- 25 mm corpus luteal cyst seen in right ovary

Explain the significance of this ultrasound report to the patient and the future management plan.

Marks will be awarded for your ability to take a relevant history, explain this report and plan the woman's further management.

Role-player's brief

- You are Mary Grant, a 35-year-old married barrister, and you have been referred by your GP for an early dating ultrasound scan, having had a positive pregnancy test.
- You have been trying for a baby for the past 5 years and this is your first pregnancy.
- You have always had a regular cycle. Your LMP was 7 weeks ago, but you have had a small amount of brown discharge for 10 days.
- Although initially delighted with the positive pregnancy test, you haven't felt pregnant for the last 4 days and you are now anxious about why the ultrasonographer would not let you see the ultrasound picture of your baby, instead asking you to see the doctor currently in the antenatal clinic.
- You have had no significant medical or surgical illnesses apart from appendicitis at the age of 15 and you are taking no medication. It is now over an hour since your original appointment time and you have a work appointment very soon in your chambers. You are concerned about the ultrasound findings but also feel pressed for time, wanting a clear and confident management plan from the doctor.
- You are quite a bossy woman and you are used to being in charge and telling everyone what to do. The doctor is much younger than you and you treat him like a student. You want answers and you want them now.

Examiner's instructions and mark sheet

History

- LMP, regular cycle
- First pregnancy
- Symptoms of pregnancy and pain
- Focused history-taking: how long has she been trying for a pregnancy
- Social history
- Date of pregnancy test being positive

0   1   2   3   4   5   6

Explanation of scan findings

- Use non-medical jargon
- This could be a delayed miscarriage
- This could be 5 weeks' gestation (re-check dates, especially pregnancy test)
- Cyst insignificant
- Explain what would be expected on scan at 7 weeks' gestation (fetal heart present)
- Check the patient has understood
- Explain that there is nothing she could have done to cause this event or prevent it
- The likelihood is that it will not happen again

0   1   2   3   4   5   6

Management

- Explain that she may ultimately require an evacuation of the uterus
- Explain the evacuation of retained products of conception (ERPC) procedure
- Offer to re-scan in a week's time and one would expect a fetal heart if pregnancy ongoing
- Offer conservative management
- Offer medical management of the missed miscarriage
- As regards the cyst, repeat ultrasound scan in 3 months if worried

0   1   2   3   4   5   6

Role-player's score

0   1   2

(2 = role-player happy to see candidate again, 1 = prepared to see candidate again, 0 = never wants to see candidate again).

Total: /20

Discussion

What does this station aim to test?

This station tests what you would normally do with an early pregnancy problem. Miscarriage is a very common problem in early pregnancy and you should be very familiar with how to deal with this problem. You should be able to take a concise relevant history, listing important points such as last menstrual period, cycle length, symptoms of pregnancy, and whether the pregnancy is wanted.

As you are dealing with a role-player, you must be sensitive to her needs, and as the management path is not clear-cut, you must be able to offer alternatives and in a way be guided by her feelings. So although you are being tested on your management skills, you are also being tested on your communication skills and it is important to check that she has understood and whether she has any further questions. This situation may well be very emotionally charged and the role-player may have been briefed to react to you in a certain way. Her occupation suggests that she is educated and may ask difficult questions.

What are the pitfalls?

You must be focused to take a concise history. Do not spend all of your time taking a thorough history as the candidate instructions advise you to take a relevant history, and explain the significance of the report and future management plans.

The corpus luteal cyst is a normal finding and you must not focus upon this as a potential problem. It is not clear-cut from the scan whether this is a viable early pregnancy of only a few weeks' gestation or whether it is a non-viable pregnancy and this must be explained to the patient. You must not be dictatorial in what you think the management should be and you must be sympathetic to what she needs. Your use of diagrams at a station such as this may be very helpful.

Your preparation

This is a very common problem that you are likely to encounter every week when you are on call. We are all at risk of becoming blasé about women who have miscarriages when we see them so often, but to the individual woman this can be a tragic event. It is also important to remember that one must use non-medical language at all times.

Prioritization on delivery suite

Candidate's instructions

> **WITH THIS TYPE OF STATION YOU RECEIVE THE INSTRUCTIONS AT A PRECEDING PREPARATORY STATION. THERE YOU WILL HAVE ADEQUATE TIME TO PREPARE YOURSELF FOR THE NEXT STATION WHERE THE EXAMINER WILL BE.**

Your instructions are as follows. You are the registrar on call for the labour ward. You have just arrived for the handover at 08.30. Attached you will find a brief résumé of the ten women on the delivery suite as shown on the board. The staff available today are as follows:

- an ST1 in her twelfth month of career training
- a third-year specialist ST3
- six midwives:
  - DB is in charge coordinator
  - DB, CD and BB can suture episiotomies
  - JR, DB and MM can insert an intravenous line.

Note: the duty consultant has been called away.

Read the board carefully. You have 14 minutes to decide what tasks need to be done, their order of priority and who should be allocated to each task.

At the next station you will meet the examiner with whom you will discuss your decisions and your reasoning.

You will be awarded marks for your ability to manage the delivery suite.

Delivery unit board (candidate's information)

Room	Name	Parity	Gestation	Liquor	Epidural	Syntocinon	Comments	Midwife
1	Barnett	1+1	32	–	Yes	Yes	LSCS at 0230 (PET) EBL 800 mL baby on SCBU	DB
2	Lawson	3+0	T+9	Mec	Yes	No	8 cm at 0300 Transferred in from home	Com/MW
3	Tifou	2+0	39	Intact	No	No	Undiagnosed breech Spont. labour 4 cm at 0730 Breech at spines	DB
4	Smith	0+0	31				Dr to see Vaginal bleeding CTG normal	BB
5	Jones	0+0	41	Mec	Yes	No	Fully at 0600	VM
6	Patel	1+0	T+2	Clear	No		Trial of scar. ARM at 0300 for VBAC FBS at 0600 pH 7.29 6 cm at 0600	JR
7	Finch	2+0	14	Intact	No	No	Routine admission for cervical cerclage	VM
8	Allpress	0+0	39				Delivered, awaiting suture	MM
9	Murphy	2+0	T+6	Intact	No	No	Spont. labour 3 cm at 0650	BB
10	Grant	0+2	32	Intact	No	No	Twins. Contracting. Ceph/ breech IVF pregnancy	MM

Examiner's instructions

The candidate has 14 minutes to explain the following:

- the tasks that need to be done on the delivery suite
- their order of priority
- the staff he/she would allocate to each.

These instructions may not be exclusive and a degree of flexibility is allowed in the marking.

Tasks required

- **Room 1** needs review after Caesarean section (CS) as the patient had severe pre-eclampsia. This review would involve pulse, blood pressure (BP), amount of ongoing blood loss, hourly urine output and fluid status. Bloods should be repeated. Medication should be reviewed.
- **Room 2** needs urgent review as she is a multiparous woman in her third labour and should have delivered by now. She has meconium liquor and has been transferred in from home so is likely to have been in labour for a very long time. Most likely malpresentation or malposition.
- **Room 3** needs urgent review to discuss mode of delivery and recommend epidural/spinal.
- **Room 4** needs assessment of the amount of bleeding, the cause and whether or not in pre-term labour. Must exclude abruption.
- **Room 5** needs review, as should have delivered by now.
- **Room 6** needs review to assess progressing adequately and review cardiotocograph (CTG) and repeat fetal blood sampling (FBS) if any CTG abnormalities.
- **Room 7** needs non-urgent review and consent to be signed after fetal viability has been checked and dating of the pregnancy has been re-checked.
- **Room 8** needs suturing.
- **Room 9** needs review later in the morning when the other cases have been sorted out.
- **Room 10** needs urgent review and appropriate assessment as may be in premature labour. If she is in premature labour, she will need steroids with tolcolysis.

The priorities for review are: room 2 is the highest priority, followed by rooms 3 and 10, and then room 4. It would be appropriate for the ST3 to see rooms 2 and 10, and the SHO to see rooms 3 and 4. The midwife could suture room 8 and room 9 could be assessed by the midwife later in the morning. After the urgent cases have been sorted out, the medical staff should review rooms 5 and 6.

Mark sheet

Room 1

0　　1　　2　　3　　4

Room 2

0　　1　　2　　3　　4

Room 3

0　　1　　2　　3　　4

Room 4

0　　1　　2　　3　　4

Room 5

0　　1　　2　　3　　4

Room 6

0　　1　　2　　3　　4

Room 7

0　　1　　2　　3　　4

Room 8

0　　1　　2　　3　　4

Room 9

0　　1　　2　　3　　4

Room 10

0　　1　　2　　3　　4

Total: /20 (divide by 2)

Discussion

What does this station aim to test?

The examiner wants to assess whether you can prioritize the problems and safely manage the labour ward. You must demonstrate an organized and confident approach and be able to defend all your decisions. Do not keep on saying that you would ask the consultant's advice, as the examiner wants to know what your decisions would be. However, clearly it would be prudent to mention that you would call the consultant and check that he or she was happy with any operative decisions. There may be different answers to this station but as long as your decisions are sensible, you'll score well.

Usually there will be 1–3 patients who will need urgent review, one to three who can be left for a while, and the rest will be those for whom the decision-making is important. You need to demonstrate to the examiner that you know what is important, that you have an organized mind and that you can hand over responsibility to other staff members, but you want to be informed of any problems they may encounter. Be clear and concise. Don't just repeat what is written on the board!

What are the pitfalls?

You cannot do everything! You must determine where you are needed the most and where the staff can go depending on their experience. You must delegate but ensure that the staff will communicate with you if further problems arise. Do not read out each room's details as it wastes time and the examiner has it in front of him/her. Give a diagnosis plus or minus a differential and explain what needs to be done, when and by whom. This is usually a high-scoring station.

Your preparation

This is an easy station to practise. Each time you walk on to a labour ward there is an OSCE station set up for you. Ideally, ask one of your seniors to spend 15 minutes with you discussing your management priorities. Practise being able to delegate duties. If you are sitting the exam at a junior level (i.e. you have never taken charge of a labour ward), ask your registrar to role-play being your junior and you do the prioritization.

Surgical skills – placenta praevia

Candidate's instructions

> **THIS IS A STRUCTURED VIVA. YOU WILL BE TESTED ON YOUR ABILITY TO APPRECIATE PREOPERATIVE, INTRAOPERATIVE AND POSTOPERATIVE MANAGEMENT OF A MAJOR OBSTETRIC PROCEDURE.**

You have admitted a 32-year-old primigravida for an elective CS. She has major placenta praevia and the presentation is breech. She is currently 38 weeks' pregnant.

The examiner will ask you five questions regarding aspects of this woman's care following her admission: counselling, preparation, techniques, postoperative care and follow-up. You will need to highlight issues related to CS in general as well as those related to this specific case.

Examiner's instructions and mark sheet

The candidate has been given the task of arranging an elective Caesarean section for major placenta praevia. Ask him/her the following questions as written.

Preoperatively what will you discuss with the patient?

- Site of placenta (anterior or posterior)
- Risks, benefits, consent
- Warn about need for IV line, catheter, possible drain, possible blood transfusion
- Type of anaesthesia and reasons
- Small risk of hysterectomy

0   1   2   3   4

What other personnel will you liaise with?

- On-duty consultant
- Anaesthetist, paediatrician, haematologist
- ODA/midwife
- Partner (warn of seriousness of operation)

0   1   2   3   4

Preoperatively what will your orders be?

- Check recent full blood count
- Nil by mouth for more than 6 hours
- Intravenous fluids, antibiotics, ranitidine, shaving, catheter, TED/Flowtron stockings
- Blood in theatre

0   1   2   3

Take me through your operative procedure and outline any concerns

- WHO checklist
- Consultant involvement
- Incision – abdominal, uterine (classical versus lower uterine), oxytocin, morbid adhesion of placenta, closure
- Quick entry through placenta and clamp cord immediately
- Be prepared for excessive blood loss

- Description of the breech delivery
- Description of closure of the uterus and abdomen

0   1   2   3   4   5

Postoperatively what would you do?

- Ensure adequate IV fluids
- Check haemoglobin
- Hourly urine output initially
- Thromboembolic deterrent (TED) stockings
- Thromboprophylaxis
- Early mobilization
- Debrief patient if necessary and discuss future pregnancies
- Contraception

0   1   2   3   4

Total: /20

Discussion

What does this station aim to test?

This woman is about to have a potentially life-threatening operation. The examiner wants to know what you would normally do before a CS as well as the extra precautions that you would take in this case. You must be thorough and go through your normal checklist, appreciating that with this type of case a lot of extra preparation is required so that the operation can be as safe as possible. The WHO checklist should be mentioned in any operative viva.

What are the pitfalls?

You must be aware of the seriousness of the case. No matter how experienced one is, this type of case can bleed excessively and be very frightening for all concerned. It is easy to miss out obvious precautions and concentrate on the more dramatic features, thus failing to carry out routine preparation.

Your preparation

Design difficult scenarios and ask your colleague to play the examiner. When a difficult surgical case occurs in your clinical practice, go back to the beginning and see whether you could have been better prepared so that the case was easier.

Communication skills – ectopic mismanagement

Candidate's instructions

The patient you are about to see has returned to the emergency gynaecology unit for follow-up after an operation for an ectopic pregnancy 14 days ago. She had a salpingostomy and the ultrasound today has shown a live ectopic on the left side.

You need to explain the results of the ultrasound scan to her, suggest management and answer her questions.

Marks will be awarded for taking a relevant history, discussing a management plan to deal with the clinical situation and addressing her concerns.

Role-player's brief

- You are Hester Greene, a 35-year-old woman who had her last menstrual period 9 weeks ago.
- This pregnancy has not been straightforward. From 6 weeks onwards you had some vaginal bleeding, and at 7 weeks you presented to the early pregnancy unit and were told that you had an ectopic pregnancy.
- You had a laparoscopy and the tube was opened up and the ectopic was removed. You were told to return the following week to check that the pregnancy levels had gone down but you didn't do this and you have continued to have some bleeding. Now you have some pain on the left side.
- When you presented today to the early pregnancy unit, they performed another scan and did another blood test. You do not know the results of the scan or the blood test, but you are just about to see a doctor who will explain the scan to you and suggest further management.
- You will be told that the ectopic remains in the left tube when you thought the operation had removed it. You are clearly very cross about this as your previous obstetric history has not been straightforward. You want to know why the pregnancy was not removed 2 weeks ago and you are now terrified that the hospital is going to make another mistake. (In your first pregnancy, from which you now have a 3-year-old child, you were originally told it was ectopic. You had a laparoscopy and it turned out to be an intrauterine pregnancy.) You are therefore adamant that you do not want them to put anything into the womb when they do a further operation until they are absolutely sure that it is a persistent ectopic pregnancy.
- You are extremely upset about what has occurred and are very cross that the pregnancy wasn't removed in the first place. You would like to see the first person who operated on you immediately so that you can express your displeasure.
- As you are now looking at a further laparoscopy, you would like conservative treatment for that tube as you do not want to rule out all possibility of a future pregnancy – your second pregnancy was a right ectopic pregnancy which was removed by laparotomy 18 months ago.
- You and your husband very much wanted this pregnancy and you are not quite sure how you are going to tell him all this bad news. You suspect that he is also going to be angry as he cares so much about you.
- You are otherwise fit and well and you take no medications and don't smoke or drink alcohol. You have no family history of any significant diseases and you are not allergic to anything.

Examiner's instructions and mark sheet

History

- Check LMP
- Check obstetric history to date
- Previous ectopic pregnancy – laparotomy
- Previous normal pregnancy originally thought to be ectopic
- Current pregnancy thought to be ectopic and had laparoscopic salpingostomy 2 weeks ago
- Failure to attend when requested
- Ask about current symptoms

0   1   2   3   4   5   6

Immediate management plan

- Explain ultrasound findings and its implications
- Needs a laparoscopy – encourage salpingectomy, however, accept her wish for conservative surgery
- Accept her wish for non-manipulation of the uterus
- Emphasize the difficulties involved and the potentially life-threatening situation

0   1   2   3   4   5   6

Future management

- Explain that persistent ectopics can occur with laparoscopic conservative surgery for tubal ectopics
- Do not blame previous surgeon for supposed negligence
- Diffuse the situation as much as possible
- Explain that in-vitro fertilization (IVF) may be the only option for future pregnancies anyway
- Contraceptive choices may be limited by her history

0   1   2   3   4   5   6

Role-player's score

0   1   2

(2 = role-player happy to see candidate again, 1 = prepared to see candidate again, 0 = never wants to see candidate again).

Total: /20

Discussion

What does this station aim to test?

This is a difficult situation where a previous operation has not been correctly performed. This station tests your ability to diffuse a situation where a woman is clearly very angry while at the same time not 'bad-mouthing' one of your colleagues. With regard to her anger, it is better to allow her to get angry at you and get it off her chest, and it is best for you to be a passive listener.

However, you do have to manage the case and you need to be quite clear in telling her what needs to be done, but you also need to accept her wish for a more conservative approach with regard to instrumenting the uterus and conservative surgery on the tubes. You also need to be quite clear that if she opts for conservative surgery again, not only is there a very small chance of the trophoblastic tissue persisting, but also, in the future, she has a further chance of an ectopic. If she was going for IVF then it is in her interests to have this tube removed.

What are the pitfalls?

It is very easy to say that the previous operation was not done correctly but you need to avoid saying this. You must take a focused history, as her pregnancy history is very important here. There are therefore three aspects to this station and one of the pitfalls is not to cover them all. You need to take a focused history, explain what needs to be done now and discuss the prognosis for future pregnancies and how you can help her.

Your preparation

These stations are difficult to prepare for because they do involve patients who are quite angry because something has gone wrong. The best way to practise this station is to ask a colleague to role-play the angry patient and to try to deflate the situation.

REVIEW STATION 6

Premenstrual syndrome

Candidate's instructions

The patient you are about to see has been referred to your outpatient clinic by her GP. A copy of the referral letter is given below. Read the letter and obtain a relevant history from the patient. You should discuss any relevant investigations and treatment that you feel may be indicated.

Dear Gynaecologist

Re: Mrs Jodie Revell aged 34 years

I would be pleased if you would see this patient who has coerced me into referring her for a gynaecological opinion. She says that she has severe premenstrual symptoms. She does not seem to have responded to anything that I have prescribed her.

Many thanks.

Yours sincerely

Dr A. Protheroe

You will be marked on your ability to take a relevant gynaecology history and discuss investigations and treatment options.

Role-player's brief

- You are Jodie Revell, 34 years old, and you are completely fed up. You have terrible premenstrual symptoms and you have been to your GP many times for this but he just tries to fob you off.
- Your main symptoms are mood swings, irritability, pelvic pain and sometimes violent behaviour. Your relationship is almost in tatters because your partner is fed up with your behaviour. You are perfectly lovely for 3 weeks out of 4, but for 7 days before your period you turn into a completely different person.
- You have had an episode of depression in the past but you don't believe that there is anything psychiatrically wrong with you. You have been violent in the past and certainly have hit your partner on numerous occasions. You have tried the odd vitamin for premenstrual syndrome (PMS) but nobody has ever really explained it to you and you are just very fed up.
- You work as an assistant to a dental surgeon and you do find it extremely stressful as the private practice is very busy. As well as working very hard, you have to be sweet and nice to everybody all of the time, otherwise your boss gets upset because his practice, and therefore his income, is also dependent on your personality.
- You had an unwanted pregnancy 6 years ago and had a termination. You are currently using the mini-pill (POP – progesterone-only pill) for contraception but you appear to have regular periods. You had Chlamydia about 3 years ago and you have been with your current partner for 5 years. It always worried you that he had strayed when you found out that you had Chlamydia.
- You have no medical or surgical history of note. You take Neurofen Extra premenstrually for the pelvic pain. You smoke 20 cigarettes a day and drink about 20 units of alcohol per week. You enjoy the odd marijuana joint and have about three per week.
- Your mother suffered from severe depression and has been on antidepressants for some years.

Examiner's instructions and mark sheet

Candidates will have 14 minutes to obtain a history relevant to the patient's complaint. They should ask about clinical examination and then investigations that they think may be relevant, explaining them to the patient along the way. They should also discuss possible treatments.

History

- History-taking to elicit the actual symptoms
- Important to establish that the symptoms are definitely premenstrual and disappear by the end of the period
- Elicit the patient's concerns about how the symptoms are affecting her home life
- Any psychiatric illnesses in the past, any family history of psychiatric illness
- Any treatments that have been tried

0   1   2   3   4   5   6

Investigations

- Explain that symptoms are related to the menstrual cycle and if not then may be some other condition
- No relevant investigations except for diary of symptoms in relation to the menstrual period

0   1   2

Management

- Validate the condition for the patient
- Emphasize that many treatments are aimed at stopping the ovulatory cycle
- Discuss management in a non-confrontational and empathic way
- Establish the diagnosis by a symptom/visual analogue diary
- Hierarchy of treatments:
  - counselling/education/reassurance/stress management and relaxation techniques
  - pyridoxine/essential fatty acids
  - selective serotonin reuptake inhibitors (SSRIs), but ensure that used specifically for PMS and not depression in this case
  - OCP/progesterone/danazol
  - oestradiol patches (or implants) plus cyclical progesterone

- gonadotrophin-releasing hormone (GnRH) analogues ± back therapy
- total abdominal hysterectomy (TAH) and bilateral salpingo-oophorectomy (BSO) followed by oestrogen hormone replacement therapy (HRT)
- Discuss the pros and cons of the various treatments
- Establish a clear plan of management including appropriate and agreed follow-up

0   1   2   3   4   5   6   7   8   9   10

Role-player's score

0   1   2

(2 = role-player happy to see candidate again, 1 = prepared to see candidate again, 0 = never wants to see candidate again).

Total: /20

Discussion

What does this station aim to test?

As with the station concerning antenatal history-taking, this station tests your communication skills and ability to take a comprehensive gynaecology history of a difficult problem. In the referral letter, the GP has stated that he was not happy to refer her on to a specialist, so there are clearly problems in the interaction between the patient and her GP. This indicates this will not be an easy consultation and you will need to be particularly good at communicating and being empathetic.

Clearly you must concentrate on her symptoms of PMS, but in a station like this it is very important that you enquire as to the effect on family, friends and work.

What are the pitfalls?

One can infer from the letter that this patient is quite desperate to receive help for her problem. She will therefore have very high expectations from the consultation and may be very emotional and have a low threshold for becoming aggressive and/or tearful. As with the antenatal history, you need to be thorough in asking about all the different aspects of history, including social and drug history, which includes recreational drugs. You should also do a systems functional enquiry. Many candidates are not organized in the way they extract information.

If the patient does become aggressive then you must defuse the situation, and at the end of the consultation you must ensure that the plan of management is clear and ask her if she has any further questions, emphasizing the next point of contact.

Your preparation

As with the antenatal history, you need to practise taking gynaecology histories and this can be easily done in pairs. Be systematic in how you take the history, as this will determine your global score in the examination.

REVIEW STATION 7

Breaking bad news – anencephaly

Candidate's instructions

You are the registrar in the Department of Obstetrics & Gynaecology. Mrs Ruth Barker, aged 28 years and pregnant for the first time, is having a scan at 16 weeks' gestation following a raised serum alpha-fetoprotein (AFP) result. The radiographer has detected that the fetus has anencephaly and has called you in, as the patient is booked under your consultant's care. You agree with her observations and have been asked to counsel Mrs Barker about these findings.

You are about to meet Mrs Barker and there is no doubt about the diagnosis. You have 14 minutes to counsel her about the situation.

You will be awarded marks for:

- explaining the diagnosis
- discussing options open to the patient
- dealing with the patient's concerns.

Role-player's brief

- You are Mrs Ruth Barker, a 28-year-old woman who has been referred for a scan because of an abnormal blood test (raised serum AFP – the spina bifida blood test) and so you have had an inkling that something is not quite right.
- It seems that all is not well, as the radiographer has called in a doctor who has suggested you discuss things in a separate consultation room. The doctor will tell you that your baby has anencephaly (the head and brain have not formed properly) and that this is incompatible with life. You will question the doctor about the options open to you, including further tests, a second opinion and the outlook for the baby if you decide to continue the pregnancy.
- You are a devout Roman Catholic and need to see your priest and partner before making any decision. You ask about the possibility of organ transplantation if you carry the baby to term.
- You are naturally upset and concerned about the possibility of future pregnancies and how you are going to cope with it mentally, whatever you do now.
- This is your first pregnancy and you have been trying to become pregnant for a few years. Otherwise you are fit and well with no family history of any significant diseases.

Examiner's instructions and mark sheet

Explaining the diagnosis

- Explain the results, avoiding jargon
- Explain that the rise in serum AFP was an indication for a scan
- Diagnosis in little doubt but can offer a second opinion
- Allow patient to express concerns, shock and confusion

0   1   2   3   4

Discussing the options

Offer options of termination or continuing pregnancy.

Termination

- Timing of termination is unlimited by the Abortion Act 1991 as the condition is incompatible with extrauterine life
- Discussion of the mechanics of the termination:
  - intracardiac potassium chloride depending on gestation
  - mefipristone tablets orally and then a series of five cervagem pessaries after 36 hours (local protocols may differ)
  - a further course may be needed if the first course does not work
  - extra-amniotic catheter if this procedure does not work
  - risk of requiring an evacuation of the uterus afterwards
  - pain relief, as the pains are similar to labour pains

0   1   2   3   4   5

Continuing with pregnancy

- Routine antenatal care would need to be undertaken
- Risk of postmaturity as fetal pituitary gland stimulates onset of labour (absent in this case)
- Difficult to get into labour as nothing pressing on the cervix
- Need for operative delivery may be necessary if shoulders are difficult to deliver or if there is poor progress in labour

0   1   2   3   4   5

Patient concerns

- Give her the option to come back after time to think it over
- Postmortem examination may be useful

- Arrange for any appropriate counselling both before and after delivery
- Consequences for a future pregnancy, recurrence rate 1 in 30
- Use of folic acid beneficial in a future pregnancy

0   1   2   3   4

Role-player's score

0   1   2

(2 = role-player happy to see candidate again, 1 = prepared to see candidate again, 0 = never wants to see candidate again).

Total: /20

Discussion

What does this station aim to test?

This station is concerned with the candidate's ability to counsel a patient and break bad news. The scenario is such that there is no doubt about the diagnosis. You need to divide your time equally between the three parts of the question. This situation is really the application of knowledge plus experience. You should appreciate that anencephalic pregnancies may progress but that there are inherent risks of postmaturity and difficulty in delivering the shoulders. It is important to provide support and not judgement; forewarned is forearmed and patients will not automatically opt for termination. A decision does not need to be arrived at by the end of the consultation. However, options need to be provided, including coming back with a partner or supporter.

The role-player will have been given the scenario. She has been given key points to test candidates' ability to apply their knowledge to the situation. If candidates are unaware of any policies then they should explain that advice would need to be sought. This approach will be reflected in the score as to how they have dealt with the situation.

What are the pitfalls?

The major pitfall in all counselling questions is that the candidate fails to read the question properly and consequently does not answer it. When in doubt candidates revert to history-taking as they feel comfortable with that. No history is required here; it is not relevant. There is no doubt about the diagnosis, but there is a tendency for candidates to give erroneous information to the role-player. It is also important to know the local protocol and apply it to the scenario. It is necessary to empathize with the role-player, but important information needs to be communicated and candidates should always be mindful of what exactly they are being asked to do, as the marking scheme will reflect those tasks.

A good candidate will be aware of the distress a diagnosis like this may cause – termination may not necessarily occur with the first course of cervagem as the patient is a primigravida, and continuation of the pregnancy is not without its risks. A good candidate is likely to draw a diagram to explain the diagnosis to illustrate the problem to the patient exactly.

Your preparation

There are three parts to this type of question and so it may be considered formulaic. The first part covers giving the diagnosis, which will not be in doubt, and the two following areas will be related to discussing the method and timing of a termination of the pregnancy or continuing it and the appropriate antenatal care that may need to be provided.

It is important, as with all the OSCEs, to utilize your time appropriately. In the examination you are given a pad to take round with you, and in this situation drawing a diagram may be a very useful way of conveying some of the information, as it can be difficult to get the role-player to take the diagnosis on board from a solely verbal explanation. It is important to remember that this news can be devastating for the patient, and one should avoid 'okay' and 'all right' and keep checking that the role-player understands the significance of what you are saying.

This station is very much the 'appliance of science', i.e. the application of your obstetric knowledge to deal with a bad news scenario. Imagine this is a clinic situation and do what you would do there. Prior to the OSCE part of the MRCOG, it would be useful to sit in with a senior as they are breaking bad news if you have no experience of doing so. It is important to allow the role-player to have time to speak as she may furnish you with valuable information. Do not be afraid of silences, provided they do not go on for too long.

What variations are possible for this question?

Breaking bad news in the obstetric scenario can be very variable, from fetal abnormality (fatal or non-fatal) to intrauterine fetal death or stillbirth. In all these scenarios there will be no doubt about the diagnosis and marks will be awarded for dealing with the situation and not for history-taking.

REVIEW STATION 8

Infertility – case notes

Candidate's instructions

THIS IS A PREPARATORY STATION.

The patient you are about to see, Susan Pesh, was referred to your outpatient clinic by her general practitioner. She was originally seen in the clinic 3 months ago and some baseline investigations were undertaken. The original notes have been lost. A copy of the original referral letter has been found, plus a copy of the original clinic letter. Copies of the results have also been placed in the notes.

You have 15 minutes to review the notes and results of the patient you will see in the next station. You will have 14 minutes with the patient to:

- discuss an appropriate supplementary history
- discuss the results of investigations
- discuss appropriate treatment options.

The Surgery
Blackhorse Road
London E44

Dear Doctor

Can you please see Susan Pesh who has a history of infertility over the past 2 years? Susan is 27 years old with a history of mild endometriosis, which was diagnosed laparoscopically 3 years ago. The endometriotic spots were found on the uterosacral ligaments only and these were diathermied. The rest of the pelvis appeared normal. Susan had been on a course of Provera for 9 months and is now asymptomatic.

Regards

Dr Twort

Dear Dr Twort

Re: Susan Pesh aged 27 years, Hosp No 707073

26 Victoria Gardens, E44

Thank you for referring this patient to my gynaecological outpatients' clinic with a history of primary infertility. She commenced her periods at the age of 13 years and appears to have a regular 28-day cycle with bleeding for 5 days. The rest of her gynaecological history is unremarkable except for a previous history of endometriosis that appears to have been successfully treated with diathermy at the time of laparoscopy and Provera. She is now asymptomatic. Her coital frequency appears to be satisfactory. Her smears are up to date. The rest of her medical history is unremarkable and she is not taking any medication.

General physical examination was unremarkable with a BP of 110/70 and a normal BMI. Pelvic examination was normal.

I have organized some routine investigations and plan to see her again in 3 months' time when the results should be available. I will keep you informed of her progress.

With best wishes

Yours sincerely

Mr A Sherman

DAY 21 PROGESTERONE (SUSAN PESH – 707073)
60 IU/L (FOLLICULAR 0–15 IU/L, LUTEAL >25 IU/L)

HYSTEROSALPINGOGRAM (HSG) (SUSAN PESH – 707073)
- The uterus is normal anteverted and mobile. Both uterine tubes fill and the isthmus and ampullary portions appear normal.
- There is free spill of contrast into the peritoneal cavity bilaterally with little retention of dye.

PELVIC USS (SUSAN PESH – 707073)
- Normal anteverted uterus, with normal looking ovaries
- No pelvic pathology seen and no evidence of PCO
- Small amount of fluid in the Pouch of Douglas (POD)

HVS RESULT (SUSAN PESH – 707073)
NORMAL COMMENSALS PLUS CANDIDA SPP.

ENDOCERVICAL SWAB (SUSAN PESH – 707073)
NEGATIVE FOR CHLAMYDIA

SEMEN ANALYSIS (BRIAN PESH, PARTNER OF SUSAN PESH)

Collection	Masturbation
Days abstinence	1 day
Time since production	90 minutes
Volume	2.8 mL
Viscosity	Normal
Motility	30%
Sperm concentration	0.6 million/mL
Abnormal form	50%
Non-sperm cell conc'n	0.3 million/mL
Total motile sperm	0.5 million
Tray agglutination test	No antisperm antibody detected

REPEAT SEMEN ANALYSIS (BRIAN PESH, PARTNER OF SUSAN PESH)

Collection	Masturbation
Days abstinence	5 days
Time since production	30 minutes
Volume	4 mL
Viscosity	Normal
Motility	35%
Sperm concentration	0.9 million/mL
Abnormal form	55%
Non-sperm cell conc'n	0.1 million/mL
Total motile sperm	2.4 million

Role-player's brief

- You are Susan Pesh, a 27-year-old woman who works as a sales assistant.
- You commenced your periods at the age of 13 years and now have a regular 28-day cycle with bleeding for 5 days. You are unsure about when you ovulate, but volunteer this information only if asked by the candidate. You have been with Brian, your husband, for 5 years and have regular intercourse, three times a week. You have been trying to get pregnant for the past 2 years.
- Apart from a laparoscopy as an investigation for pain on intercourse you have had no other surgical procedures. You were treated for mild endometriosis, although you are a little unsure about the nature of it. The rest of your history is unremarkable. Your last smear was prior to your referral and the result was normal. You have used the oral contraceptive pill in the past but at the age of 21 for 9 months only.
- You are a non-smoker and you are not taking any medication.
- Your partner is likewise fit and well and works as a panel beater. He is a non-smoker and drinks a glass of wine with meals. He does, however, like to smoke marijuana at least once a week. He has not had any previous testicular problems and has not fathered a child.
- You are getting anxious and depressed because all your family are expecting you to get pregnant as easily as your two sisters and all your school friends are on at least their second baby by now.
- The results would suggest that there is a male factor and so the candidate should explain the various technologies available to you. You feel your partner may get very distressed at the thought that it is probably his problem and not yours.

Examiner's instructions and mark sheet

Appropriate supplementary history

- May ask about LMP
- May ask if partner has had any testicular problems, tumours, infections, operations
- Ask about history of smoking, alcohol and any recreational drugs
- May ask about type of underwear and bathing habits
- Any previous children from either partner
- May check about coital frequency
- May ask about Candida and whether she has had treatment or is still symptomatic [wrong name on result sheet]

0   1   2   3   4   5   6

Discussion of investigations and relevance

- Ovulating normal midluteal progesterone
- Fallopian tubes patent on the HSG
- Infection status negative for Chlamydia but positive for Candida [wrong name on result sheet]
- Semen results show main problem is with a low sperm count
- Further count may be useful but diagnosis is unlikely to be different
- Candidate notices wrongly labelled results for candida

0   1   2   3   4   5   6

Discussion of appropriate treatment options

- Never say that the patient can never get pregnant, but may have difficulties
- Advise to stop marijuana, usual advice about underwear, baths and multivitamins
- Advise that intrauterine insemination (IUI) may not be very successful
- Donor insemination may not be the first line of treatment
- Suggest reproductive technologies IVF/ICSI
- NICE guidelines suggest IVF should be available on the NHS and she would appear to be eligible
- Ask patient how far she wants to proceed, and say adoption may be an option

0   1   2   3   4   5   6

Role-player score

0   1   2

Total: /20

Discussion

What does this station aim to test?

This has a preparatory station in order to allow the candidate to read the case notes. However, it could be placed at the station to go through with the patient present, which would simulate what can happen in reality.

The question looks at whether the candidate can interpret the clinical findings and results. This is the kind of scenario in which one may find oneself in a clinic with very basic information and copies of letters. It is unlikely that there will be a role-play couple. You may have to counsel either the woman or her partner in this kind of a situation. It could be the man who you are seeing to discuss his sperm count and this may lead to a very confrontational consultation. The actors will have been primed to ask specific questions in order to lead you along the score sheet of the examiners.

There are three aspects to what is required and it is important to think of relevant questions related to the low sperm count. With all infertility questions, there will usually be an obvious diagnosis. It is always important to find out how far along the road of assisted treatments a couple is prepared to go.

The examiner will be in place to award marks and nothing else.

What are the pitfalls?

The major pitfall is in answering the question, being critical of the notes and allowing yourself time to deal with all three tasks. This is clearly a case of infertility due to a male factor. It is important that the candidate has a clear idea of the normal values of the common tests that are undertaken in the gynaecological outpatient clinic. In most cases the normal ranges will be given, but even so the candidate should know the normal range of any test requested. This is particularly true in obstetrics when the normal range may change due to the pregnancy.

As in real life, it is important to check that the results belong to the patient in front of you. There may be results that have been deliberately labelled incorrectly and these need to be identified. This is especially true if you are breaking bad news.

Your preparation

There are three parts to this question. In the preparatory station it is worth making notes of specific parts of the history that have not been addressed or documented to date. These would revolve around any possible reasons for a low sperm count, such as drugs, history of previous children, and other social issues. The second part of the question is to interpret the results to the patient, and that can be done only if normal values are known. The third part of the question is to discuss the low sperm count and the specific options that may be useful for this case. You would need to have a clear idea about the options and how to get access to them.

It is important in all fertility patients to check their LMP as they may already be pregnant.

What variations are possible for this question?

Alternatives to this scenario would be endocrinology cases where a number of results are given to the candidate and those results have to be interpreted to the gynaecologist. As the examination may occur over 2–3 days, comparable stations will need to be found for each day.

REVIEW STATION 9

Audit

Candidate's instructions

A copy of an algorithm that is used in the early pregnancy assessment unit is supplied. This protocol was instituted in an attempt to reduce the number of unnecessary ultrasound scans performed.

Discuss with the examiner how you would design an audit to ascertain how well this protocol is being adhered to, and what steps you would take if the audit revealed that overall compliance was poor. You are not being asked to comment on or criticize the protocol as such.

You will be awarded marks for:

- discussing the factors you would take into consideration
- designing an audit to address the question
- discussing how you would use the results.

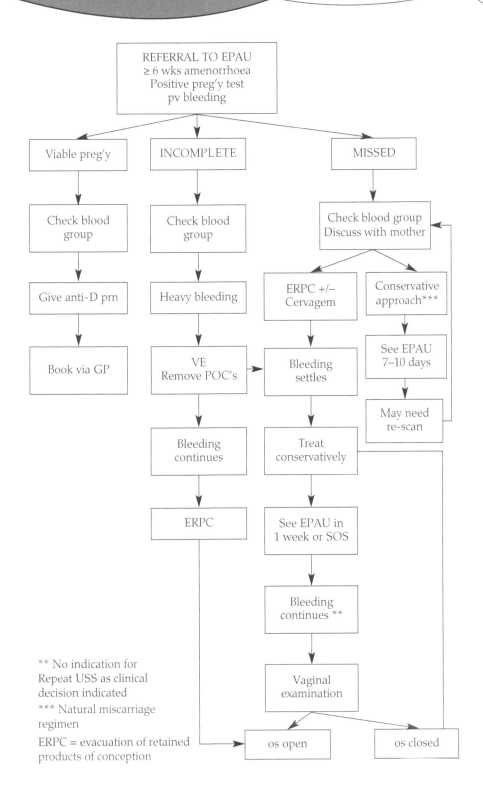

** No indication for
Repeat USS as clinical
decision indicated
*** Natural miscarriage
regimen
ERPC = evacuation of retained
products of conception

Examiner's instructions and mark sheet

Candidates need to cover the following areas of discussion and can be prompted by a specific question if they do not mention them spontaneously.

Factors to be considered

- Which patients should have been managed?
- Evidence-based medicine
- RCOG/national guidelines
- Consumer interaction/expectations
- Previous complaints
- Previous audit findings
- Encouraging all stakeholders to make comments

0   1   2   3   4   5   6

Design the audit

- Determine sample size
- Establish a data sheet/proforma to identify patients' course
- Define outcome criteria
- Identify missing data and eliminate bias
- Identify key failures in following the algorithm
- Should the audit be prospective or retrospective and the inherent problems in both

0   1   2   3   4   5   6

Use of results

- Feed results back to staff; may need to talk to GPs or hold stakeholder meetings
- Anticipate reactions
- Hard on the issue, soft on the individual: avoid a blame culture
- Consider any necessary organizational changes to improve or allow compliance
- Resource implications for change
- How to achieve consistent implementation involving the stakeholders
- Decide when audit should be repeated
- Time taken for changes to be implemented
- Change in protocol may not make further audit comparable
- Completing the audit cycle

0   1   2   3   4   5   6   7   8

Total: /20

Discussion

What does this station aim to test?

This station is designed to test the candidate's understanding of audit. The algorithm or protocol is relatively immaterial. It is not the protocol that is being criticized but the adherence to the protocol that is being tested. There may be a preparatory station prior to meeting the examiner. The examiner will expect the candidate to go through the steps of an audit cycle. If the examiner has to prompt the candidate then the marking will be reflected accordingly.

What are the pitfalls?

The major pitfall in this type of question is not understanding the audit process and spending the time criticizing the protocol. All UK trainees are expected to undertake some form of audit during their postings and this is the place to learn how to do it. You need to be aware of proforma or data sheets that need to be produced and whether the audit should be done on a numbers basis or over a specified time. That will reflect the frequency of the condition. For early pregnancy problems, it may be useful to do the next 200 cases; if the subject was water births then it may be worth using a fixed time period instead. Most audits should be done prospectively as there is a risk of losing cases retrospectively, which may alter the ultimate outcome.

Your preparation

The following is a way of undertaking an audit. It is useful for a candidate to have undertaken an audit within his or her own organization.

- Agree audit scope and objectives
- Audit methodology/design
- Review current practice
- Agree preferred practice
- Design proforma/audit tool
- Collect data
- Analyse data
- Conclusions/recommendations
- Action plan
- Re-evaluation

Obstetric history

Candidate's instructions

The patient you are about to see has been referred to your antenatal clinic by her GP. A copy of the referral letter is given below. You have 14 minutes to read the letter and obtain a relevant history from the patient. You should discuss any relevant investigations that you feel may be indicated. The GP's examination of the patient should be taken to be unremarkable.

You will be awarded marks for:

- obtaining an obstetric history
- establishing risk factors for this pregnancy
- discussing relevant and appropriate investigations.

The Surgery
High Street
Enfield

Dear Doctor

Would you please book Ms Rollings for antenatal care? She is 11 weeks pregnant. I have enclosed some of the investigation results.

Yours sincerely

Dr Beattie

INVESTIGATIONS (ANDREA ROLLINGS AGED 30 YEARS)

- FBC – normal
- Blood group – O, Rh-negative, no antibodies
- VDRL – negative
- Rubella – non-immune
- Mid-stream urine (MSU) – no growth
- USS – single live intrauterine pregnancy consistent with 11 weeks' gestation, no other abnormalities detected

---

Role-player's brief

- You are Andrea Rollings, a 30-year-old woman who works in the sex industry. You are single and live alone.
- Your periods are regular every 28 days with a 5-day bleed. You had been using the oral contraceptive pill but this pregnancy was due to a pill failure. You are unsure of the date of your last menstrual period and don't see it as relevant when you know that the recent scan makes you 11 weeks pregnant.
- This is your first pregnancy and you have a certain amount of ambivalence towards it. You are also off-hand with anyone you see as an authority figure. You don't make the interview easy, as you view the doctor in this way.
- Your personal/medical information is as follows:
  - Medical and surgical history – nothing noteworthy
  - Last cervical smear was 5 years ago
  - Smoke 20 cigarettes a day
  - Drink alcohol, about three units a day
  - Use recreational drugs – marijuana and cocaine (but no intravenous usage)
  - Medication and allergies – none.

Examiner's instructions and mark sheet

Familiarize yourself with the candidate's instructions and the role-player's brief. Candidates should discuss with the patient any relevant investigations they feel are appropriate. Investigations that need to be considered by the candidate are:

- hepatitis B and C screen
- HIV test
- cervical smear
- HVS and *Chlamydia* swabs.

Obstetric history

- Basic obstetric history, including LMP, cycle length, expected date of delivery (EDD)
- Medical and surgical history and any family history of note
- Is it planned and does she want to continue with the pregnancy
- Occupation and deals with social factors, looking at alcohol, cigarette, recreational drug consumption and domestic violence
- How the pregnancy is progressing to date

0   1   2   3   4   5   6

Risk factors

- Brings out the fact that she may be at risk of HIV and substance abuse
- How she is supporting her habits
- Ask about occupation
- Emphasize the importance of attending for routine antenatal check-ups
- Patient is not immune to rubella, which may not be a problem at this stage of the pregnancy but would recommend immunization after the pregnancy
- Patient is Rhesus negative and will need appropriate administration of anti-D and antibody checks during the pregnancy
- History of any sexually transmitted diseases
- Discussion of risks of cocaine on the pregnancy

0   1   2   3   4   5   6

Relevant investigations

- Routine investigations done, including FBC, group, rubella, syphilis
- Discussion about Down's screening
- HIV screening

- Cervical cytology
- *Chlamydia* testing and HVS should be considered
- Hepatitis B and C
- Detailed scan at 20 weeks

0   1   2   3   4   5   6

Role-player's score

0   1   2

(2 = role-player happy to see candidate again, 1 = prepared to see candidate again, 0 = never wants to see candidate again).

Total: /20

Discussion

What does this station aim to test?

This station tests the ability of the candidate to take a basic obstetric history and, in so doing, establish the risks for this patient and her pregnancy. Once the correct questions have been asked, any relevant investigations and appropriate management should ensue. It is looking at a patient who has a high risk of sexually transmitted disease, risk of an abnormal smear and also the possibility of drug abuse and the problems that may ensue in a pregnancy.

The GP's examination is taken to be normal and so there should be no interaction with the examiner, whose role is to mark according to the prescribed mark sheet. The role-player has been given a scenario and will answer questions when asked. She will have been briefed as to how much help to give candidates and in some cases will have specific questions to ask candidates in order to help them with the questions. If the question does not have a bearing on the scenario, the role-player will answer that all is normal.

What are the pitfalls?

The major pitfall in an obstetric history-taking station is that, in the UK, a midwife takes most full obstetric histories so the candidate does not routinely take a history. Key points are therefore not covered, such as whether this was a planned pregnancy, occupation, menstrual history and smear history.

A lot of antenatal care involves routine screening and it is important to appreciate this fact when it comes to taking a history. It is important to elicit risk factors, including tobacco and alcohol consumption. It is important to ask about recreational drugs, and it is best asked in those terms.

As with any pregnancy, a plan of action needs to be formulated and a decision arrived at as to whether the pregnancy is high-risk or low-risk.

Another major pitfall that arises in many of the role-playing stations is the use of medical jargon, and especially abbreviations. The role-players are not medical personnel (to simulate a real clinic setting), and they may not understand medical terms. They may pick you up on this – which can be very disconcerting and throw you off balance at a stressful time for you.

Your preparation

This particular patient may seem to be a 'nightmare patient', but it is important to go back to the instructions as to what is required. Get into the habit of taking routine obstetric histories and formulating plans for the pregnancy in the 14 minutes allocated. It is also useful to go through booking notes in the antenatal clinic to assess risk factors.

Most history-taking questions are relatively straightforward, although in an OSCE situation there may be some kind of twist in the story. The role-player may have been primed to ask questions to steer you along a certain track.

Finally, be aware of the screening blood tests that are done routinely in the UK.

Breaking bad news

Candidate's instructions

> **THIS IS A COUNSELLING STATION.**

You are the registrar in the gynaecological outpatient clinic and you are about to see Ms Kay Trench, a 39-year-old single woman who underwent a hysteroscopy and curettage 2 weeks ago and is here to obtain the results. She has had a history of heavy, irregular vaginal bleeding for the past 6 months and was treated by her GP with a course of oral contraceptive pills (OCPs) with no relief. She was subsequently referred to this hospital for further investigation. Below is the histology report. Please counsel Ms Trench.

Four Mills District Hospital, Leicestershire
Department of Pathology

Patient name: Kay Trench
ID no.: T7785254
Age: 39
Date: 28 December 2010

Specimen: uterine curettings

Histology report
Moderately differentiated adenocarcinoma of the endometrium

Validated by:

_____

Dr Nisha Khan
MRC Path.

You will be awarded marks for the following:

- your ability to take a relevant history
- your explanation of the diagnosis
- your explanation of the patient's subsequent management and concerns.

Role-player's brief

- You are Ms Kay Trench, a 39-year-old primary school teacher.
- You are single, not sexually active and will be married to your fiancé, Richard, in 6 months. You love children and plan to have three.
- You currently live with your parents and three brothers and you are close to your family.
- Your first period (menarche) was at age 10. Your periods are irregular with each cycle lasting 1–6 months. Your periods last 4–5 days and are not heavy. You have mild, tolerable dysmenorrhoea. You have always thought this pattern of periods was normal.
- You have never used contraception and have never had a cervical smear.
- You have not taken any regular medication except in the last 3 months.
- You have not noticed any weight change but have always been chubby. You have not noticed any increased hair growth.
- You do not smoke, and drink alcohol socially on occasions.
- Six months ago your periods suddenly became frequent, occurring every few days, and heavy with clots. There has been no associated abdominal pain.
- Your GP prescribed a course of the combined OCP for the past 3 months. The medication reduced the flow of the periods but there was still daily vaginal spotting.
- You were then referred to this hospital for a hysteroscopy and dilation and curettage (D&C). You are well following the D&C. There are no abdominal pains or vaginal discharge but you continue to have daily vaginal spotting.
- You are worried about the result of the operation.
- You are extremely upset about learning of the cancer, especially when you are to be married and plan to have children.
- You are suspicious that your GP has treated your symptoms conservatively for 3 months, making a difference to the stage of the disease now.

Prompt questions

- What is the result of the operation, doctor?
- Is it cancer? Is it curable? Why has this happened to me?
- Is there no way for me to have children in the future?
- What are the risks of the surgery?
- What are the risks and side-effects of radiotherapy?
- Why didn't my GP refer me earlier – I may not have developed cancer?

Examiner's instructions and mark sheet

Familiarize yourself with the candidate's instructions and the role-player's brief. Do not award half marks.

Relevant history

- Menstrual history – previous irregular, long cycles, never took medication except the OCP in the last 2 months
- Risk factors – no diabetes mellitus, non-smoker, non-drinker, nulliparous
- No family history of any cancers
- Fertility desires – to be married in 6 months, wants to have children
- Social support – financially stable, good family support, good relationship with parents and siblings
- No medical/surgical history

0   1   2   3   4   5

Explanation of histology report

- Malignancy of lining of womb
- Extent of disease unknown; will need staging, which is surgical
- Will need MRI and discussion of both imaging and pathology at a multidisciplinary team (MDT) meeting to decide further management
- Need for total hysterectomy and bilateral salpingo-oophorectomy, possible lymph node dissection
- Surgery procedure – GA, midline incision; risks of surgery, i.e. anaesthetic risks, venous thromboembolism, bladder, bowel injury, bleeding, infection
- Possible laparoscopic assisted vaginal hysterectomy (LAVH) depending on MDT findings

0   1   2   3   4   5

Discussion of consequences of treatment

- No further fertility, menopause and consequent risk of osteoporosis, climacteric symptoms
- Risk of HRT is likely to be low
- Prognosis depends on staging; varies from 85 per cent in stage 1 to 10 per cent in stage 4 in 5-year survival
- May need postoperative radiotherapy, depends on histology
- Once diagnosis given, then 31-day target to commence treatment.

0   1   2   3   4   5

Counselling

- Addresses patient's concern about GP's initial conservative management
- Offers counselling to cope with news
- Answers role-player's remaining questions

0   1   2   3

Role-player's score

0   1   2

(2 = role-player happy to see candidate again, 1 = prepared to see candidate again, 0 = never wants to see candidate again).

Total: /20

Preoperative ward round

Candidate's instructions

You are the registrar responsible for today's operating list. Your consultant will be in the hospital but has an important meeting and would prefer not to be disturbed. You now have to do the preoperative ward round. There are three patients on the list:

1 Mrs Andrews – a 42-year-old for a total abdominal hysterectomy
2 Mrs Devine – a 33-year-old for a diagnostic laparoscopy
3 Mrs Norman – a 35-year-old for a resection of a submucosal fibroid

You are about to meet the examiner. He/she will ask you some questions about what you would normally do with each patient preoperatively. You have 14 minutes during which you should answer the examiner's questions.

Examiner's instructions and mark sheet

Please ask the candidate the following questions as they are written. Do not prompt and do not award half marks.

1 Mrs Andrews is a 42-year-old woman with a 20-week fibroid uterus for a total abdominal hysterectomy.

- What relevant history do you want to know?
  - What are her main symptoms
  - Does she have any menopausal symptoms
  - Has she received any GnRH analogues
  - Any previous surgery, especially abdominal
  - Has subtotal hysterectomy been discussed

0   1   2   3   4

- What investigation results would you like to know?
  - USS findings
  - Any available endometrial histology
  - Full blood count (FBC)
  - Pregnancy test
  - Cervical smear

0   1   2   3   4

- What other aspects of the procedure would you discuss with her?
  - Does she understand what operation she is having
  - Confirm ovarian conservation has been discussed
  - Discuss incision: vertical may be necessary
  - Risks of complications, namely haemorrhage, bowel/bladder damage
  - Need for thromboprophylaxis

0   1   2   3   4

- What would you warn her to expect postoperatively?
  - Catheter
  - IV line
  - Possible need for a drain depending on intraoperative blood loss

0   1   2

- Is there anything else you would consider doing before checking her consent form?
  - Examine her abdomen
  - Ask if she has any questions

0   1   2

2 **Mrs Devine** is a 33-year-old woman who is having a laparoscopy for right-sided pelvic pain (? endometriosis).

- What relevant history do you want to know?
  - Nature of pain
  - How long she has had the pain
  - Exact site of pain
  - Obstetrics and gynaecology (O&G) history
  - Past surgery

0   1   2   3   4

- What investigation results would you like to know?
  - USS findings
  - FBC
  - Pregnancy test
  - Cervical smear

0   1   2

- What would you discuss with her before she signs the consent form?
  - Does she know what operation she is having
  - If endometriosis is found, diathermy or excision would be useful

0   1   2

- What would you warn her of?
  - Bowel/bladder trauma
  - Where the skin incisions will be

0   1   2

- Is there anything else you would consider doing before checking the consent form?
  - Examine her abdomen
  - Ask if she has any questions

0   1   2

3 **Mrs Norman** is a 35-year-old woman who has a 3 cm diameter submucosal fibroid that has been causing her regular periods to be heavy.

- What relevant history do you want to know?
  - Any O&G history
  - Any previous surgery

0   1   2

- What results of investigations would you like to know?
  - FBC
  - USS findings
  - Pregnancy test
  - Cervical smear

0   1   2   3   4

- What would you check she has had preoperatively?
  - GnRH agonists

0   1

- What intraoperative complications would you warn her of?
  - Uterine perforation which would then require a laparoscopy and possibly further surgery
  - Possible risk of requiring a laparotomy if complications occur

0   1   2

- Anything else you would consider doing before checking her consent form?
  - Examine or inspect her abdomen
  - Ask if she has any questions
  - Discuss the need for thromboembolic deterrent (TED) stockings and possible thromboprophylaxis, depending on the length of the procedure

0   1   2   3

Total: /20 (score divided by 2)

Obstetric history and management

Jacqueline Tyler, the patient you are about to see, has just been admitted to your maternity unit. The midwife is concerned about her and no other doctor is available to see her at present. You have 14 minutes to obtain a history from the patient and outline the plan of management.

> **THIS STATION TESTS YOUR ABILITY TO TAKE AN OBSTETRIC HISTORY AND YOUR COMMUNICATION SKILLS WITH REGARD TO MANAGEMENT.**

You will be awarded marks for:

- taking an obstetric history
- discussing a relevant management plan for the patient.

Role-player's brief

- You are Jacqueline Tyler and you are 39 years old. This is your second pregnancy and you have reached 26 weeks' gestation: last menstrual period (LMP) = 26 weeks earlier; expected date of confinement (EDC) = 14 weeks later.
- This pregnancy is the result of in-vitro fertilization (IVF) + intracytoplasmic sperm injection (ICSI) (third attempt) after 5 years of infertility due to severe problems with the quality of your partner's sperm.
- Your first pregnancy was at the age of 17 years and you had a termination at 10 weeks' gestation.
- You booked at the maternity hospital at 12 weeks' gestation.
- You had a nuchal translucency test at 12–14 weeks and this gave you a Down's syndrome risk of 1 in 200.
- Chorionic villus sampling at 12 weeks was uneventful. Result: normal male karyotype.
- Detailed ultrasound scan at 20 weeks was normal.
- The day before admission you felt generally unwell (feverish, tired). Several hours prior to admission you experienced a gush of fluid vaginally and there has been persistent vaginal dampness since.
- You are now aware of lower abdominal cramps.
- Personal – married, secretary.
- Mother has insulin-dependent diabetes mellitus (IDDM).
- One sister has spina bifida, another sister had a deep vein thrombosis (DVT) while on the OCP.
- You do not smoke, drink less than 5 units of alcohol per week and do not use recreational drugs.
- Drugs taken – folic acid.
- Medical history – congenital dislocation of the hip (CDH) as a baby, and have had subsequent recurring hip problems.

Role-player's attitude

You are very worried about your situation and fear that you are going to lose your baby. You continually seek reassurance from the doctor.

Examiner's instructions and mark sheet

Familiarize yourself with the candidate's instructions and the role-player's brief.
Do not award half marks.

History

- Personal details
  - termination of pregnancy at 10 weeks' gestation
  - age
- Family history
  - IDDM
  - NTD
  - DVT
- Social history – non-smoker
- Menstrual history
  - CDH
  - Infertility

0   1   2   3   4

Presenting complaint

- Gestation LMP/EDC
- Premature prelabour rupture of membranes (PPROM)
- Contraction-type pains and their nature
- Sequence/timing

0   1   2   3   4

Current pregnancy

- IVF + ICSI
- Nuchal translucency test result
- Chorionic villus sampling (CVS) and result
- Detailed ultrasound scan result
- Any medication

0   1   2   3   4

Management

- Advise admission
- Speculum examination to confirm rupture of membranes
- Steroids for lung maturity

- Initial scan for liquor volume, growth
- Monitor WBC, C-reactive protein (CRP)
- Cardiotocograph (CTG), though can be difficult to interpret sometimes in premature pregnancies
- Expectant management
- Antibiotics

0   1   2   3   4

Neonatal management

- The baby is likely to be delivered early and will require paediatric involvement
- May require transfer to the tertiary unit
- Outcome will depend on the weight and maturity of the baby

0   1   2

Role-player's score

0   1   2

(2 = role-player happy to see candidate again, 1 = prepared to see candidate again, 0 = never wants to see candidate again).

Total: /20

Management problem – gynaecology

Candidate's instructions

A 40-year-old nulliparous social worker, Ms Tracy Sumner, has been referred to you by her GP complaining of painful heavy periods. She bleeds for 10 days every month and has so much pain that she is sometimes bedridden for the first two days of her period. She has had regular cervical smears, all of which have been normal.

Four years ago she had a lumpectomy for breast cancer and is now on tamoxifen. She smokes 20 cigarettes a day and is otherwise well. She is fed up and wants something done. She has tried medical therapy.

You have examined her and found:

- BMI = 30 kg/m^2
- Soft, obese, distended abdomen
- 24-week-sized irregular abdomino-pelvic mass, confirmed to be fibroids on ultrasound scan – posterior fundal fibroid ($12 \times 10 \times 10$ cm); submucosal fibroid ($3 \times 4 \times 4$ cm).

You are about to meet Ms Sumner. You have 14 minutes to take a relevant history and then outline the management options open to her and their attendant risks.

You will be awarded marks for:

- taking a relevant history
- discussing the procedures open to the patient
- outlining the risks of those procedures

Role-player's brief

- You are Ms Tracy Sumner, a 40-year-old social worker.
- For the last 3 years you have had very heavy periods, bleeding for 10 days every month, and the pain throughout the periods can be unbearable. You even go to bed during the first two days of your period when the pain is so bad.
- Periods are regular.
- You have been told that your womb is enlarged and sometimes you feel that there is pressure on your bladder as you have to pass urine frequently.
- You have never tried to get pregnant as you still have not met the right man. You have had partners in the past but none at the moment. You accept that you may not get pregnant and will consider a hysterectomy.
- You have tried all sorts of tablets and nothing has helped the bleeding. You tried the mirena (an IUCD with progesterone in it) but felt ghastly on it so had it removed after 3 months. You are at the end of your tether and want something done about it.
- Your general health has been good, but 4 years ago you had breast cancer and had a lumpectomy, and you have been taking tamoxifen since surgery.
- You have had regular Pap smears, which were normal.
- You smoke 20 cigarettes a day as you have a very stressful job.
- You are allergic to amoxil (you get a rash).
- There is a family history of ovarian cancer (mother and maternal aunt).

Examiner's instructions and mark sheet

Familiarize yourself with the candidate's instructions and the role-player's brief. Do not award half marks.

Enquiries about the relevant history

- O&G history – nulliparous
- Other treatments that have been tried
- Is she in a stable relationship
- Is fertility an issue
- Any pressure symptoms regarding bladder or bowel
- Has she had a recent blood count
- Recent cervical smear test

0   1   2   3   4

Which surgical procedure (need endometrial biopsy first)?

- Hysteroscopy – resection of submucosal fibroid/endometrial ablation if no fibroid – unlikely to be effective with such a large uterus
- Myomectomy – open procedure
- Subtotal hysterectomy ± BSO
- Total abdominal hysterectomy ± BSO
- Other options:
  – arterial embolization
  – do nothing

0   1   2   3   4

Risk of procedures

Immediate

- Anaesthetic – GA risks
- Bladder/bowel injury
- Haemorrhage
- Risk of unwanted hysterectomy (for hysteroscopy and myomectomy)

Intermediate

- DVT/PE
- Bladder problems
- Infection

Long term

- DVT/PE
- Bladder problems
- Psychosexual, including loss of womanhood if ovaries removed

0   1   2   3   4   5

Advantages and disadvantages of procedures

- Hysteroscopy – less invasive but may need further procedure as pressure symptoms won't be improved
- Myomectomy – will preserve fertility but must understand chance of hysterectomy and massive bleeding (fertility is probably limited as she is 40 years old with no current partner)
- Subtotal hysterectomy (or total abdominal) – both may induce premature menopause; subtotal is the easier operation, there are fewer bladder problems postoperatively and possible better sexual function; however, cervix remains – potential site of cancer, possibly may still bleed
- Other options are still in the research arena.

0   1   2   3   4   5

Role-player's score

0   1   2

(2 = role-player happy to see candidate again, 1 = prepared to see candidate again, 0 = never wants to see candidate again).

Total: /20

Prenatal counselling

Candidate's instructions

You are the registrar in the antenatal clinic. Ms Anna Reid, a 35-year-old Caucasian woman, has been married for the past year and is planning her first pregnancy. She is keen to find out more about genetic testing for cystic fibrosis (CF). Please counsel Ms Reid.

> **THIS IS A COUNSELLING STATION.**

Marks will be awarded for the following:

- taking a relevant history from the patient
- providing an explanation of CF
- discussing the risks for a baby affected by CF
- discussing the management options for the patient.

Role-player's brief

Profile

- You are Ms Anna Reid. You are 35 years old, married for the past year and are now keen to start a family. You have never been pregnant.
- You are Roman Catholic by religion.
- A few months ago your mother revealed to you that you had a brother who was affected with CF and passed away at age 6 years, before you were born.
- Your periods are regular, normal flow, no dysmenorrhoea. Your last cervical smear was 12 months ago and was normal. You have not used any form of contraception.
- You have no medical/surgical history of note.
- Your husband, Alan, is aged 40 and is a Caucasian. He is Protestant by religion.
- As far as you know, his family has no history of CF.

Your concerns about the disease

- You are worried about the possibility that any child you conceive may be affected with CF.
- You would like to know more about the disease.
- You would like to know whether you are a carrier.
- You would like to know whether the disease can be detected in the baby and how it can be tested.
- You would like to know the accuracy of testing.

Examiner's instructions and mark sheet

Relevant history

- Age, parity and religion – 35 years old, para 0, Roman Catholic
- Family history – mother has revealed to her that she had a brother who was affected with CF before she was born and passed away at age 6
- No medical/surgical history of note
- Husband's age and race – aged 40 and a Caucasian
- History of CF in husband's family – none of note

0   1   2   3   4

Explanation of the disease

- Inherited disease, inherited in an autosomal recessive manner
- Affects lungs, digestion and reproduction
- Basic problem is in the production of mucus and saliva, which leads to recurrent chest infections, indigestion and malnutrition
- Intelligence is normal
- Chronic condition requiring prolonged care and multiple hospital visits
- Life expectancy is to the twenties or thirties

0   1   2   3   4

Risks of her baby being affected

- A child is affected if he or she inherits one affected gene from each parent and has two abnormal genes.
- With the history of her brother being affected, Ms Reid is either normal with no affected genes or is a carrier with one affected gene.
- If she and her husband are both carriers, then the risk of the baby being affected is 25 per cent. The risk of the baby being a carrier is 50 per cent and the baby has a 25 per cent chance of being normal.

0   1   2   3   4

Genetic testing

- In a Caucasian population, the chance of a person being affected is 1 in 25.
- Parental testing can be done to determine whether a person is a carrier.
- Genetic testing identifies up to 90 per cent of all CF gene mutations but may miss 10 per cent of mutations.

- Testing whether the baby is affected allows the parents to know whether the pregnancy is affected and, if so, allows termination of the pregnancy if they are not prepared to care for such a child.
- Fetal testing can be done by testing the baby's cells via one of two methods – amniocentesis or chorionic villus sampling.

0   1   2   3   4   5   6

Role-player's score

0   1   2

(2 = role-player happy to see candidate again, 1 = prepared to see candidate again, 0 = never wants to see candidate again).

Total: /20

Obstetric emergency – uterine inversion

Candidate's instructions

You are the registrar in charge of the labour ward. You are urgently called by the midwife. She has just discovered that a patient who had a vaginal delivery has collapsed.

You arrive in the room and the midwife is there with the uterus inverted and placenta attached.

The examiner will ask you a series of four questions about the management of this patient.

> **YOU WILL BE MARKED ON YOUR ABILITY TO ANSWER THESE QUESTIONS FROM THE EXAMINER WITH REGARD TO THE EMERGENCY OUTLINED.**

Examiner's instructions and mark sheet

Familiarize yourself with the candidate's instructions and then ask the following four questions as written.

What will be your immediate management actions on being faced with this case?

- This is an obstetric emergency and the candidate should go to see the patient immediately.
- Activate emergency code to mobilize SHO, anaesthetist and midwife.
- Establish and maintain this woman's airway and begin chest compression if patient is asystolic. An intravenous line should be started and blood for FBC, coagulation profile, U&E and creatinine levels, group and save should be taken.

0   1   2   3   4

What will be your subsequent management of this patient?

- Place patient in lithotomy, clean and drape and catheterize.
- Prompt gentle replacement of the uterine inversion manually – last-out/first-in method.
- Use of uterine relaxant such as terbutaline 0.25 mg IV, or general anaesthesia in the operating theatre.
- Hydrostatic method (O'Sullivan's method) – the inverted uterus is held within the vagina and warm saline infused (about 2 L is infused rapidly into the vagina).
- If still unsuccessful, may need emergency laparotomy and replacement of uterus by traction on round ligaments.
- As a last resort, a Caesarean hysterectomy may be necessary.
- Once stable, correction of anaemia or coagulopathy with blood and fresh frozen plasma, if necessary.
- Use of oxytocin drip should be started to maintain uterine contractility.
- Observation in high-dependency unit for hourly BP, heart rate and urine output measurements.
- Antibiotic cover should be started.
- Placenta should be removed at some stage unless thought to be morbidly adherent.

0   1   2   3   4   5   6

What other steps would you take in the management of this patient?

- Inform duty consultant.
- Inform the patient's partner or next of kin and warn them of preventive steps at next delivery, i.e. controlled cord traction with fundal guarding in the third stage of labour.
- May need to discuss the mode of delivery in a subsequent pregnancy if she has been traumatized by the event.
- Record the events systematically and chronologically in the case notes.
- Record the events in an 'incident report' form.
- Arrange a follow-up appointment.

0   1   2   3   4   5   6

What risk management issues are important here?

- Incident form needs to be completed
- Review by risk management team
- Team advise update on management of third stage protocol
- Audit how often it happens
- Disseminate results

0   1   2   3   4

Total: /20

Operating list prioritization

Candidate's instructions

> **THIS IS A PREPARATORY STATION**

You are asked to go through a consultant's gynaecology waiting list and advise the waiting list manager on:

- appropriate procedure(s) (operation and others)
- venue of proposed treatment (outpatient department, day unit, inpatient)
- special needs (if any)
- priority of assignment – routine (18 weeks from referral), urgent (within 4 weeks), target (31/62-day cancer target rule), or emergency (immediate admission).

You have 15 minutes to consider these cases before meeting the examiner to describe your actions and offer explanations wherever appropriate. You will be awarded marks for your ability to manage and prioritize the cases.

Waiting list for operations (candidate's information)

Name	Age	Details	Operation and logical action	Venue	Special needs	Priority
JA	28	Deep dyspareunia; menorrhagia; ovarian cyst (4 cm, scan suggests benign)				
AB	42	Large pelvic mass; likely ovarian cyst, CA125 = 45 IU/mL				
JF	18	Recent abnormal smear; cervical biopsy; CIN3; requests treatment under GA				
PH	30	P3+1; recent TOP; history of subacute-bacterial endocarditis and DVT; wants laparoscopic sterilization				
PR	18	Primary amenorrhoea/cyclical pain; ultrasound shows distended vagina				
KR	32	P5+0; missing IUCD; caring for invalid child (IUCD in abdominal cavity)				
QT	44	Fibroid uterus; menorrhagia; haemoglobin 8.1; Jehovah's Witness				
TN	82	Recent angina (failed pessary); procidentia/lives alone/incontinent				
TL	28	Pelvic pain; previous laparotomy (twice)				
JB	22	Secondary subfertility – 3 years; previous ectopic				

Examiner's information

Waiting list for operations

Name	Age	Details	Operation and logical action	Venue	Special needs	Priority
JA	28	Deep dyspareunia; menorrhagia, ovarian cyst (4 cm, scan suggests benign)	Hysteroscopy and laparoscopy ± mirena Laparoscopic cystectomy	Day unit		Routine
AB	42	Large pelvic mass, likely ovarian cyst, CA125 = 45 IU/mL	Refer to MDT for surgical recommendation; laparoscopy or laparotomy; consultant must be present	Inpatient	MRI MDT review	Target
JF	18	Recent abnormal smear; cervical biopsy; CIN3; requests treatment under GA	Large loop excision of transformation zone (LLETZ)	Day unit	Within NHSCSP guideline target	Urgent
PH	30	P3+1; recent TOP; history of subacute-bacterial endocarditis and DVT; wants laparoscopic sterilization	Laparoscopic clips sterilization	Day unit	ECHO cardiogram then NICE guidelines if need for prophylactic antibiotics Appropriate thrombo-prophylaxis	Routine
PR	18	Primary amenorrhoea/cyclical pain; ultrasound shows distended vagina	Incise hymen	Day unit		Urgent
KR	32	P5+0; missing IUCD; caring for invalid child (IUCD in abdominal cavity)	Laparoscopy? Proceed laparotomy	Inpatient, but home same day if possible	Good notice Bowel prep	Urgent

QT	44	Fibroid uterus; menorrhagia; haemoglobin 8.1; Jehovah's Witness	Abdominal hysterectomy	Inpatient	Check recent Hb: oral iron GnRH analogues	Routine
TN	82	Recent angina (failed pessary); procidentia/lives alone/incontinent	Vaginal hysterectomy and repair needs	Inpatient	Arrange postop care Preoperative assessment ECG Chest xray Exclude possibility or recent infarct	Urgent
TL	28	Pelvic pain, previous laparotomy (twice)	Laparoscopy (excision of endometriosis if present)	Inpatient	Warn of risk of bowel damage	Routine
JB	22	Secondary subfertility – 3 years; previous ectopic	Laparoscopy dye, hysteroscopy, possible endometrial biopsy	Day unit	Check ovulation Check sperm count	Routine

Examiner's instructions and mark sheet

Discuss each case briefly, and mark each case globally. If there are ten cases then score each out of 4, and divide the overall score by 2. If there are eight cases then score each out of 5, and divide the overall score by 2.

Total: /20

Extra notes

The answers are not clear-cut so one needs to confirm that there is a common-sense approach.

- AB: It should be clear that a consultant must be present for this operation.
- KR: This operation might be successfully done laparoscopically but if this proves impossible, a laparotomy may be necessary. The operative arrangements should reflect this, so it may be best to admit her as an inpatient on the understanding that, if a laparotomy proves unnecessary, she might go home on the same day. The special needs arrangement for the care of her invalid child would have to reflect the 'worst' scenario. Does she need the operation at all?
- QT: The operation could include either TAH or subtotal hysterectomy (not myomectomy). The candidate should discuss the preoperative treatment of the anaemia and the prerequisite of a normal blood count prior to surgery. Although oral iron may be sufficient, the discussion should also include hormonal ovarian suppression if this fails. The special operation consent form is best done prior to admission.
- TN: The use of anaesthetic preoperative assessment should be discussed.
- TL: This patient is best admitted as an inpatient because of the possibility of bowel damage during laparoscopy. She should be warned of this risk.
- JB: Is this appropriate? Will need Chlamydia screening and prophylaxis.
- JA: Check Ca125.
- PH: Mirena inserted under antibiotic cover may be a safer option.

Bereavement

Candidate's instructions

Mrs Tina Shoe was a 26-year-old primigravida who presented to the labour ward with a 24-hour history of decreased fetal movements at 39 weeks' gestation. At that time her general observations were normal. The fetal heart could not be heard and an intrauterine fetal death was confirmed by ultrasound scan.

The pregnancy had been classed as 'low risk' and antenatal care was provided by the community midwife and GP. Mrs Shoe had considered a home delivery. She was a bit of a worrier and had experienced some abdominal pain 24 hours prior to admission. At that time she had a CTG performed in Triage which was reported as normal. Consequently she had been sent home. The CTG was subsequently reviewed and considered to be suboptimal.

Following the diagnosis of fetal demise, labour was induced and after 12 hours Mrs Shoe delivered a 2.3 kg macerated stillborn male infant with the cord wrapped tightly around the neck. The patient's postnatal course was a little stormy, as her blood pressure was quite labile, rising to 140/100 mmHg with 2+ proteinuria. This settled after 36–48 hours.

At this station you will meet Mrs Shoe's husband, who has turned up on the labour ward to see you 2 weeks after the event. His wife is physically well but has gone to stay with her mother in Bournemouth. The husband is very angry and is demanding an explanation for the death of his son.

Postmortem has shown an anatomically normal male infant weighing 2.3 kg. All fetal and maternal investigations were normal.

Marks will be awarded for your ability to deal with a difficult situation and to counsel an angry bereaved person as well as answering his questions.

Role-player's brief

You are Mr Shoe and work as a window cleaner. You are at your wits' end. Your wife has had a stillborn and she blames herself for it. She is a worrier and continued to smoke throughout the pregnancy but only 10 cigarettes a day. She has had to go to her mother's house, as she cannot cope at home when you are out at work. This event has put a real strain on the marriage and you feel she may never try for a baby again in case the same thing happens. Certainly sex is out of the question at the moment so you have to relieve yourself and you are getting fed up with it.

You cannot understand how this happened as the pregnancy had been considered low risk and you had even thought about a home delivery. You want to know if the midwife and GP did not provide the appropriate care. The baby seemed very small and you can't understand why that wasn't picked up – after all, your wife seemed to be down at the antenatal clinic for hours at a time. Why hadn't she had more scans?

Prompts for questions/remarks

- 'Why did this happen when she had some monitoring the day before and the doctor at that time said everything was all right?'
- 'Who is to blame and what are you going to do about it?'
- 'I'm going to complain and go to the papers. This shouldn't happen in this day and age. I am going to sue this hospital.'
- 'I want to see the boss man.'

Examiner's instructions and mark sheet

Familiarize yourself with the candidate's instructions and the role-player's brief. Do not award half marks.

Communication skills

- Appropriate introduction
- Sympathetic approach – not responding aggressively
- Expression of sympathy
- Allowing husband to talk – not interrupting
- Asking about his wife and how they are coping as a couple
- Maintaining eye contact
- Trying to defuse anger – allows the role-player to vent his anger

0   1   2   3   4   5   6

Dealing with the case

- Recognizing IUGR
- Fetal demise may have been due to intrauterine growth restriction (IUGR) which may have been PET-induced
- Cord around fetus may be causal or incidental
- Explanation of postmortem findings, avoiding medical jargon
- Advice for future pregnancy, including aspirin, folic acid, serial scans

0   1   2   3   4   5   6

Advice/comments

- Not incriminating colleagues
- Not becoming agitated at mention of legal action
- Explain access to complaints procedure (Patient Advice and Liaison Service – PALS)
- Offer to meet again with his wife and the carers
- Offer to discuss management in a further pregnancy

0   1   2   3   4   5   6

Role-player's score

0   1   2

(2 = role-player happy to see candidate again, 1 = prepared to see candidate again, 0 = never wants to see candidate again).

Total: /20

.

Emergency contraception

Candidate's instructions

The patient you are about to see has attended the gynaecological ward for emergency contraception. She is Ruth Hale and is 31 years old. You are the registrar on call and the staff on the ward would like you to see her as they are short-staffed and, owing to bed shortages, the ward is full of elderly patients. The staff are very busy and unable to deal with this patient unless she waits a considerable time. You have 14 minutes to deal with her.

Marks will be awarded for:

- taking an appropriate history
- counselling her appropriately
- discussing appropriate examinations.

Role-player's brief

- You are Ruth Hale, a 31-year-old librarian. You live at home with your aged parents but were coerced into going out on a hen party last night. You got a bit drunk and became quite disinhibited. Your friends set you up with a blind date at the party, which was held in one of your colleague's houses. One thing led to another and you had unprotected intercourse with him. This is unusual behaviour for you as you have had only one sexual partner in the past, and that was soon after you finished university.
- Your last period was 2 weeks ago, your cycle is usually about 28–30 days and you usually bleed for 5 days. You have never had any pregnancies or gynaecological problems in the past. You do, however, suffer intermittently from migraines. You have no known allergies and are not taking any medication.
- It is now about 12 hours since you had intercourse and you are still a little hung over and also disinhibited, so may be a bit crude and graphic about what happened.
- You do not feel you could cope with the embarrassment of being pregnant at this stage in your life, although you would love to become pregnant at some stage.

Prompts for questions

- 'What methods are there?'
- 'What is the failure rate?'
- 'What happens if it fails, would it affect the baby?'
- 'You won't have to examine me will you?'
- 'This is confidential isn't it?'

Examiner's instructions and mark sheet

Familiarize yourself with the candidate's instructions and the role-player's brief. Do not award half marks.

History

- LMP and check it was normal
- Patient's menstrual cycle
- Calculate date of ovulation
- Has not had sex for many years
- Days in the cycle of unprotected sex
- Number of hours since episode of unprotected sex
- Current method of contraception
- Any potential contraindications

0   1   2   3   4   5   6

Counselling

- Methods available, mode of action and risks
- Levonelle × 2, 12 hours apart, or IUD time limit 5 days
- Failure rate and implications
- Attitude to possible pregnancy if the method fails
- Importance of follow-up
- Discuss what she needs to do if the method fails
- Make final decision about postcoital contraception (PCC)
- Warn about action if vomiting occurs (if within 2 hours with Levonelle then take second dose and get a repeat prescription)
- Discuss contraception in current cycle
- Long-term contraception needs
- Keep accurate records, time and date
- Discuss STD screening

0   1   2   3   4   5   6   7   8

Vaginal examination

- May reveal concealed pregnancy
- May reveal possible infection
- Do microbiological swabs (though may be too early)
- IUD suitability

0   1   2   3   4

Role-player's score

0   1   2

(2 = role-player happy to see candidate again, 1 = prepared to see candidate again, 0 = never wants to see candidate again).

Total: /20

CIRCUIT A, STATION 10

Intermenstrual bleeding

Candidate's instructions

The patient you are about to see has been referred to your outpatient clinic by her GP. A copy of the referral letter is given below. You have 14 minutes to read the letter and obtain a relevant history from the patient. You should discuss with the patient any relevant investigations and management options that you feel may be indicated.

The Surgery
Lauriston Road
Hackney
London E9

Dear Doctor

Re: Hetty Buckingham aged 34 years

Would you please see this patient who seems to have been getting some intermenstrual bleeding (IMB) over the last 12 months. She has a BMI of 23 and pelvic examination was normal and, in particular, the cervix looked normal.

Yours sincerely

Dr A.P. Rilfool MRCGP

You will be awarded marks for:

- taking a relevant history
- discussing appropriate investigations
- discussing appropriate management options.

Role-player's brief

- You are Hetty Buckingham, a 34-year-old accountant in a stable relationship. You have a 4-year-old son who was a normal delivery and he weighed 3.2 kg.
- You have been on the OCP (microgynon) for many years and it has always suited you. You were recently diagnosed as epileptic and started on some medication for this condition. You are vague about the epilepsy and mention it only if asked. You are currently taking carbamazepine 200 mg daily. You have noticed recently that you have become a bit forgetful and occasionally forget to take the odd OCP.
- You and your partner are not keen on a further pregnancy.
- You have noticed over the past 3–6 months that you have had some IMB but no postcoital bleeding. Your periods are otherwise regular every 28 days, bleeding for 4–5 days. You are otherwise well and asymptomatic. There is no history of note except for some degree of irritable bowel syndrome.
- You also want to explore with the doctor some other form of contraception. You are unsure of your last smear test (both the result and when it was performed).

Examiner's instructions and mark sheet

History-taking

- Length IMB occurs in cycle
- Any postcoital bleeding
- Elicits history of epilepsy
- Carbamazepine
- Wants to consider other contraception

0   1   2   3   4   5   6

Investigations

- Do another pelvic examination to do a cervical smear and exclude any local pathology
- Arrange an ultrasound scan
- Blood test may not be necessary unless other indications in the history

0   1   2   3   4

Management

- Discusses fact that OCP may not be high enough dose with carbamazepine

0   1   2

- Discusses either:
  - Increasing the dose of OCP – may not want to change the pill or may want a different type of contraception, may consider progesterone-only pill (POP) and the possible problems
  - IUCD
  - Mirena
  - Depoprovera/implanon
  - Sterilization

0   1   2   3   4   5   6

Role-player's score

0   1   2

(2 = role-player happy to see candidate again, 1 = prepared to see candidate again, 0 = never wants to see candidate again).

Total: /20

Labour ward prioritization

Candidate's instructions

You are the registrar on call for the delivery unit. You have arrived for the handover at 8.00 am. Attached you will find a brief summary of the 10 women on the delivery suite as shown on the board.

The staff available today are as follows:

- an obstetrics and gynaecology ST2, in post for 6 months
- a third-year anaesthetic registrar (ST3)
- the on-call consultant has been asked to deal with a labour ward patient who was transferred to the intensive care unit (ICU) during the night
- six midwives: SW is in charge; SW, CK and MC can suture episiotomies; DB, SW and PL can insert intravenous lines.

Read the board carefully. You have 15 minutes to decide what tasks need to be done, in which order they should be done, and who should be allocated to each task. You will then meet the examiner to discuss your decisions and your reasoning.

Marks will be awarded for:

- your ability to manage each case
- prioritizing each case
- delegating the most appropriate staff to deal with each case.

Candidate's information

Rm	Name	Para.	Gest.	Liquor	Epid.	Synt	Comments	Midwife
1	Marsh	1	39	Intact	No	No	Undiagnosed breech; contracting 1 in 4; just admitted and VE – cervix effaced and 5 cm dilated	PL
2	Ford	2	41	Intact	No	No	Spontaneous labour; 6 cm at 3 am	IND, MW
3	Hammond	0	20	Membranes intact	No	No	Cervagem TOP for hypoplastic left heart; stopped contracting at 7 am; review ? for oxytocin	CK
4	Khan	5	39	Clear	No	No	Contracting — spontaneous labour; 7 cm at 7 am; ? urge to push	MC
5	Grantham	0	33	Membranes intact	No	No	Readmitted with APH at 2 am; no contractions; CTG normal	CK
6	Chan	1	T+10	Intact	No	No	For induction of labour for post dates; prostaglandin gel inserted midnight	MC
7	Hodgkins	0	39	Intact	No	No	Contracting; 4 cm at 4 am; repeat VE at 7 am still 4 cm	VM
8	Adams	0	39	–	–	–	Delivered at 6 am; awaiting sutures	SW
9	Bryant	3+1	39	–	No	No	For elective CS (2 previous CS)	VM
10	Ngosa	1	38	Meconium	Yes	No	Spontaneous labour; contracting 1 in 3; CTG suspicious; pH at 7.30 am was 7.23, cervix 7 cm	DB

Examiner's instructions

The candidate has a total of 14 minutes to explain to you his or her ability to:

- manage each case
- prioritize each case
- delegate the most appropriate staff to deal with each.

EACH CASE SHOULD BE MARKED GLOBALLY:
0 = POOR; 1 = SATISFACTORY; 2 = AVERAGE; 3 = GOOD;
4 = EXCELLENT.

The following is a guide for marking each case globally.

Room 1 – Marsh

- *Tasks*. Needs an emergency Caesarean section (CS), intravenous line insertion, taking full blood count (FBC) and group & save. May need a repeat vaginal examination (VE) if it looks as though she is progressing quickly. Will need a consent, VTE thromboprophylaxis assessment.
- *Priority*. Urgent
- *Personnel*. Registrar (self)

Room 2 – Ford

- *Tasks*. Needs artificial rupture of membranes (ARM) ± syntocinon. Check her urine for ketones. May need intravenous fluids. Need to know why she is not fully dilated. Check the fetal heart and that there are no underlying problems. Possible malposition.
- *Priority*. Semi-urgent
- *Personnel*. SW (coordinator)

Room 3 – Hammond

- *Tasks*. Needs assessment to see whether gestational sac is sitting in the vagina, which may need manual removal of pregnancy or further course of cervagem.
- *Priority*. Semi-urgent
- *Personnel*. Registrar (self)

Room 4 – Khan

- *Tasks.* Needs VE to assess whether fully dilated and allow to deliver. Will need IV line and active third stage as she is a grand multip. If not fully dilated consider analgesia. Check there are no fetal concerns.
- *Priority.* Urgent
- *Personnel.* Midwife MC

Room 5 – Grantham

- *Tasks.* She will need an assessment to see whether she is in labour. Check recent ultrasound scan to look for placental location and growth. Check venflon in situ. Review notes to check her cervix has been visualized to exclude a local cause. Has she had steroids as this is a readmission? Ensure the neonatal unit is aware and can accept the baby if she needs delivery.
- *Priority.* Routine (unless other information given about deteriorating picture)
- *Personnel.* ST2

Room 6 – Chan

- *Tasks.* Needs a repeat VE. Further prostaglandin or ARM if possible. Will need cardiotocograph (CTG). Defer until emergency Caesareans are concluded.
- *Priority.* Routine
- *Personnel.* Midwife MC

Room 7 – Hodgkins

- *Tasks.* Needs ARM ± syntocinon. Recommend IV fluids, exclude ketonuria. Likely to be either occiput posterior (OP) or occiput transverse (OT) position. May benefit from an epidural.
- *Priority.* Semi-urgent
- *Personnel.* Midwife VM

Room 8 – Adams

- *Tasks.* Needs suturing – should have been performed within an hour of delivery which is a target for labour ward. Check not bleeding excessively.
- *Priority.* Semi-urgent in view of time of delivery
- *Personnel.* Midwife SW

Room 9 – Bryant

- *Tasks.* Check consent, recent FBC, group & save, MRSA swab result.
- *VTE assessment.* Check when she last ate and drank.
- *Priority.* Routine
- *Personnel.* ST2

Room 10 – Ngosa

- *Tasks.* Needs repeat fetal blood sampling (FBS) if not apparently ready to deliver. Further action will depend on that result. May need to expedite delivery. Check CTG: may need group & save.
- *Priority.* Urgent
- *Personnel.* Registrar (self)

Mark sheet

SCORE GLOBALLY

Room 1

0   1   2   3   4

Room 2

0   1   2   3   4

Room 3

0   1   2   3   4

Room 4

0   1   2   3   4

Room 5

0   1   2   3   4

Room 6

0   1   2   3   4

Room 7

0   1   2   3   4

Room 8

0   1   2   3   4

Room 9

0   1   2   3   4

Room 10

0   1   2   3   4

Divide scores by 2:

Total: /20

Abdominal pain – premature labour

Candidate's instructions

The patient you are about to see is Kylie James and she has just been admitted to your maternity unit. The midwife is concerned about her and, as the labour ward registrar on duty, you are asked to assess Ms James.

You have 14 minutes to obtain a history from the patient. Seek information relevant to her current pregnancy, determine the reason for her admission, and formulate a management plan.

Examination reveals a normal temperature and blood pressure but her pulse rate is about 90 beats per minute. The dipstick test of her urine is normal. On abdominal palpation, the uterus is equivalent to her dates with a breech presentation. There is no tenderness but the uterus appears irritable. On VE the cervix is effaced but not dilated with the presenting part at the level of spines and intact membranes. An obstetric calculator is supplied.

You will be awarded marks for your ability to:

- take a relevant history from the patient
- make a provisional diagnosis
- formulate a management plan.

Role-player's brief

- You are Kylie James. You have an uninterested attitude and are awkward to the point of being obstructive.
- You are 21 years old. This is your second pregnancy, which has reached 29 weeks.
- This pregnancy is unplanned, resulting from a casual relationship and failed barrier contraception. Your previous pregnancy was terminated at 8 weeks as you were then 15 years old and still at school.
- Last menstrual period (LMP) – date of exam minus 29, giving appropriate expected date of delivery (EDD).
- You booked at the maternity unit at 16 weeks.
- All the antenatal blood tests were normal as far as you can remember.
- Antenatal care has been provided by your midwife as you don't like hospitals.
- An ultrasound scan at 20 weeks showed a normally grown fetus equivalent to your dates. The ultrasonographer noted the presence of a choroid plexus cyst. You were seen by the consultant and reassured. Rescan at 24 weeks did not show any choroid plexus cyst.
- The day before admission you had felt generally unwell with intermittent crampy abdominal pains. However, during the night you developed abdominal pains that were more regular and are now lasting about 30 seconds every 4–5 minutes. You have also had some vaginal discharge that is slimy and bloodstained.
- You are single, unemployed and live at home with your parents, three brothers and two sisters. You are the eldest and it does get a bit crowded from time to time.
- Family history – your mother is a non-identical twin.
- You smoke 20 cigarettes a day, and drink alcohol at the weekends (6–7 bottles of lager), depending on the cashflow situation. You have no idea what you are going to do when the baby arrives, with regard to accommodation.
- Drugs – occasional ecstasy tablet but not since you found out you were pregnant. You have never used any drugs intravenously. You use inhalers (becotide and ventolin) for asthma when necessary but not on a regular basis.
- You keep asking the candidate: 'What is the cause of the pain?'

Examiner's instructions and mark sheet

Familiarize yourself with the candidate's instructions. The candidate is asked to:

- take a relevant obstetric history
- make a diagnosis
- formulate an appropriate management plan.

Score the candidate's performance on the mark sheet. The role-player will have a maximum of 2 marks to award the candidate. You should not interact with the candidate, and do not give half marks.

History

Presenting complaint

- Asks about the nature of her pain, radiation and any precipitating factors
- Contractions – sequence and timing
- Any vaginal bleeding, discharge or loss of liquor

Current pregnancy

- Age
- LMP/EDD
- Unplanned
- Type of care
- Scan results regarding choroid plexus cyst
- Blood test results

History

- Obstetric previous termination of pregnancy (TOP)
- Social history and situation
- Cigarette and alcohol intake
- Drugs, both therapeutic and recreational use
- Family history that may be relevant
- Medical history
- Any previous sexually transmitted diseases

0   1   2   3   4   5   6   7   8

Provisional diagnosis

- Preterm labour most likely diagnosis
- Investigate cause – may need to send off mid-stream urine (MSU), FBC and C-reactive protein (CRP)
- Fibronectin test and explain to the patient the indications and value of it
- Infection elsewhere in the body needs to be excluded
- Differential diagnosis including urinary tract infection (UTI), appendicitis, concealed abruption or bowel problems (though most unlikely with the evidence given)
- May benefit from an ultrasound scan to assess size and confirm presentation of fetus

0   1   2   3   4   5

Treatment plan

- Patient needs admission; discuss aims of treatment to prolong the pregnancy
- Try to stop contractions with ritodrine/atosiban according to department protocol
- Intramuscular steroids to reduce the severity of respiratory distress syndrome
- Discuss with the neonatal unit as to cot availability, inform the paediatricians (she may require transfer to a tertiary unit)
- Mode of delivery needs to be considered if she goes into labour properly

0   1   2   3   4   5

Role-player's score

0   1   2

(2 = role-player happy to see candidate again, 1 = prepared to see candidate again, 0 = never wants to see candidate again).

Total: /20

CIRCUIT B, STATION 3

Urinary incontinence

Candidate's instructions

The patient you are about to see was referred to your outpatient clinic by her GP. A copy of the referral letter is given below. You should accept the GP's examination findings as correct.

You have 14 minutes to read the letter and obtain a relevant history from the patient. You should discuss with the patient any relevant investigations and treatment that you feel may be indicated.

The Surgery
Pines Lane
Newhampton

Dear Doctor

Please see Mrs Martha Gray who is a part-time learning support assistant and who has been experiencing urinary symptoms for 4–5 years. These have mainly been urgency and frequency but she has recently been 'wetting herself' and feels that the children think she smells.

She can feel a lump coming down in the vagina which is affecting her lifestyle.

She is overweight and her current body mass index (BMI) is 32, though she has lost some weight recently. General physical examination was normal, but she has a moderate cystourethrocele. A recent cervical smear test was normal, and an MSU showed *E. coli*.

Please see and treat as required.

Yours sincerely
Dr Beattie

You will be awarded marks for:

- obtaining a relevant history from the patient
- discussing relevant investigations
- discussing appropriate management options.

Role-player's brief

- You are Martha Gray, a 56-year-old woman, who works as a part-time schoolteacher. Your main problems are as follows:
  - urinary frequency, passing urine 8–10 times a day
  - passing urine at night (nocturia), 2–3 times a night, but no bedwetting
  - when you've got to go, you've got to go, with occasional accidents of not getting to the toilet on time
  - leaking when you cough, laugh, sneeze and run for a bus, and so you do not do much exercise to try to reduce your weight as it is too embarrassing
  - occasional stinging on passing urine.
- You went through the menopause at age 48 years, with no gynaecological problems. You have had three children, all normal deliveries and all weighing over 4 kg. You remain sexually active.
- The rest of the history is unremarkable, although you smoke 15–20 cigarettes a day and seem to be always 'chesty'.
- You are overweight but claim not to eat very much at all, and you have lost 4 kg recently. You drink at least 10 cups of tea/coffee a day and have a 'cuppa' just before going to bed.
- Whenever the doctor suggests investigations, you need to ask exactly what they involve. Ask about how the bladder pressure studies are performed and why they are undertaken.

Examiner's instructions and mark sheet

Familiarize yourself with the candidate's instructions. The candidate is asked to:

- take a relevant obstetric history
- discuss relevant investigations
- discuss appropriate management options.

Score the candidate's performance on the mark sheet. The role player will have a maximum of 2 marks to award the candidate. You should not interact with the candidate, and do not give half marks.

Relevant history

- Age
- Basic urinary symptoms – frequency, nocturia, urgency, dysuria
- Incontinence history and any enuresis
- Basic gynaecological history including date of LMP, smear history and whether still sexually active
- Obstetric history, deliveries and size of babies
- Fluid intake, especially quantity and timing of tea/coffee (i.e. caffeine intake)
- Family and social history, including smoking
- Occupation and how it affects her work
- Check about her weight situation and exercise levels

0   1   2   3   4   5   6

Relevant investigations

- Repeat MSU to ensure it has been adequately treated
- Random blood sugar, or possibly a fasting one; if concerns, may need a glucose tolerance test
- Urodynamics: need to explain what is done with a catheter in the bladder, transducer in the rectum and filling the bladder and looking at the voiding. Not dignified but not painful. Need to ensure MSU negative before undertaking it. The aim is to give a diagnosis as to the stability of the bladder.

0   1   2   3   4   5

Management options

- Recommend continued weight loss and stopping smoking
- Refer for physiotherapy and pelvic floor exercises (60 per cent of cases may notice improvement)
- May benefit from HRT if tissues atrophic
- Treat UTI if still present
- May need to manage non-insulin-dependent diabetes if indicated by blood glucose levels
- Reduce fluid intake, especially caffeine intake; advise on timing of intake to reduce nocturia; may be useful to keep a fluid diary for a few days to get the message home
- See in 3 months for review
- May offer ring pessary to see if it improves her feeling of a lump in the vagina before her next visit

0   1   2   3   4   5   6   7

Role-player's score

0   1   2

(2 = role-player happy to see candidate again, 1 = prepared to see candidate again, 0 = never wants to see candidate again).

Total: /20

CIRCUIT B, STATION 4

Prioritization of GP letters

THIS IS A PREPARATORY STATION.

You are a year 3 specialist registrar (SpR) and your consultant's secretary has asked you to prioritize some letters from the local general practitioners to the most appropriate clinic. You have 15 minutes to read the letters and outline your plan for each referral as follows:

- nature of the presenting complaint
- allocation of each case to the most appropriate clinic
- prioritization of each case
- suggest any additional investigations that should be done prior to the patient's visit in order to enhance the patient journey
- give reasons for your comments.

You will meet the examiner to discuss the cases at the next station.

LETTER 1

Dear Doctor

Re: Ms AB, aged 34 years

Would you please see this patient who has recently joined our practice? She attended for routine cytology screening. She is from Lithuania and her English is limited. The cervical test result shows:

Severe dyskaryosis, please refer to Gynaecologist.

She has had three full-term normal deliveries, but no other history of note.

Please see and advise.

Yours sincerely

Dr Smith

LETTER 2

Dear Doctor

Re: Miss CD, aged 66 years

Would you please see this single woman who presented with a history of vaginal bleeding and discharge over the past few weeks? She is currently on warfarin for her atrial fibrillation (AF). She lives alone and, apart from the AF, she doesn't have any other medical problems, though her BMI is 32.

She has never been sexually active so I decided not to examine her as it wouldn't alter my need for referring her.

Yours sincerely

Dr Jones

LETTER 3

Dear Doctor

Re: Ms EF, aged 32 years

Would you please see this 32-year-old woman who has been in her current relationship for 4 years? She has been trying to get pregnant for the past 2 years. Her menstrual periods are regular. She has had one previous suction TOP when she was a student. She was subsequently on the oral contraceptive pill for more than 10 years. She has not had any medical problems in the past. She is a non-smoker and is not currently taking any medication except for folic acid.

Her last cervical smear was earlier this year and it was negative.

Many thanks

Yours sincerely

Dr White

LETTER 4

Dear Doctor

Re: Ms GH, aged 44 years

I would welcome your further opinion on this 44-year-old woman. She has had polycystic ovary syndrome (PCOS) in the past but now presents with a 3-month history of heavy irregular bleeding. When she bleeds, she passes blood clots and has episodes of flooding. In view of her age I thought that she probably needs the expertise of a gynaecologist.

Her other problem is morbid obesity and she has now developed non-insulin dependent diabetes. She is currently on metformin and is a moderate smoker (despite my best efforts at trying to get her to stop).

She has had a smear this year though it was back-breaking trying to visualize the cervix.

I remember your comments about these types of patient at the recent menstrual disorders seminar you did for us local GPs.

Thanks for seeing her and good luck.

Best wishes

Dr Hope

LETTER 5

Dear Doctor

Re: Ms IJ, aged 38 years

I would like you to see this 38-year-old ICU nurse who came for a cervical smear test. I had difficulty visualizing the cervix and so did a VE to check it wasn't retroverted. On examination she had a swelling in her pelvis that extends up to her umbilicus. Her pregnancy test was negative.

On questioning she appears to have some pressure symptoms of urgency and frequency but no pain. I think this is likely to be a big fibroid uterus. She is extremely keen to preserve her fertility. She has been on the internet and would like to discuss conservative approaches to her problem. She is generally fit and well with no significant medical history and she is on no medications.

Yours sincerely

Dr Brown

LETTER 6

Dear Doctor

Re: Ms KL, aged 60 years

I would be pleased if you could see this patient who presents with a 6-month history of urgency and occasional incontinence and a lump in her vagina. She has a history of emphysema though has had a good year to date.

Her BMI is normal but the symptoms she is getting severely restrict her social activities, which is upsetting her as she has just retired and wants to make the most of her retirement.

Yours sincerely

Dr Mitchell

LETTER 7

Dear Doctor

Re: Ms MN, aged 25 years

This patient attended for her first cervical smear test today. She is nulliparous with regular periods and no gynaecological or medical history of note. She is currently using Yasmin as contraception and it has been suiting her until lately when she has been getting some postcoital bleeding.

When I took her smear today, there was a lot of bleeding when I had finished. I am not sure whether this was just due to an erosion or whether she had a polyp.

I would be extremely grateful for your help.

Best wishes

Yours sincerely

Dr James

LETTER 8

Dear Doctor

Re: Ms OP, aged 32 years

I would be grateful if you would see this patient who has some sort of menstrual disorder. She was on the oral contraceptive pill until a year ago as she is keen to start a family. However, she is getting pain with intercourse so it is not all that frequent. She also has problems with heavy periods.

I haven't examined her vaginally as she had a normal cervical smear test performed about 9 months ago.

Best wishes

Yours sincerely

Dr Worth

LETTER 9

Dear Doctor

Re: Ms ST, aged 67 years

I wonder if you would see this patient who has had a 12-month history of vulval itching. I have tried some HRT and Canesten to no avail. She is very independent and currently looks after her mum who is 99 years old.

She declined examination today but I have explained that someone will look at her vulva when she attends.

Yours sincerely

Dr Bridge

LETTER 10

Dear Doctor

Re: Ms WY, aged 22 years

I would be grateful if you could see this 22-year-old woman who presented earlier this month to discuss contraception. I took off some blood just to check her hormones as she mentioned that her periods had become very light and less frequent. Prolactin at that time was significantly increased. On the advice of the lab this was repeated 3 weeks later when not only had the prolactin increased further but the follicle-stimulating hormone (FSH) and luteinizing hormone (LH) had now been significantly suppressed (results enclosed).

I am embarrassed to say that I haven't a clue as to what is going on with this woman. She has no obvious medical condition and is on no medications, apart from the contraceptive pill which she commenced after her first visit and before we had received the results of her blood tests.

Yours sincerely

Dr A Martin

Results	Normal	Date 1	Date 2 (+23 days)
LH (U/L)	2.5–9.0	12.4	<0.5
FSH (U/L)	3.0–9.0	5.1	<0.5
Prolactin (mu/L)	60–500	2487	3997

Examiner's instructions

Familiarize yourself with the candidate's instructions, the referral letters and the tabulated case summaries below. Each referral should be marked globally on the candidate's justification for his or her answers.

These are the candidate's instructions:

- Determine the nature of the presenting complaint
- Allocate each case to the most appropriate clinic
- Prioritize each case
- Suggest any additional investigations that should be done prior to the patient's visit in order to enhance the patient journey
- Give reasons for your comments.

The final global score should take into consideration the candidate's ability to demonstrate:

- clinical competence and awareness
- ability to organize and prioritize the clinical scenario.

Case summaries (examiner's information)

Highlighting presenting problem	Additional investigations	Clinical priority
1. Severe dyskaryosis may have major grade lesion	May need interpreter	2-week colposcopy wait (NHSCSP guidelines)
2. Postmenopausal bleeding	Needs scan for endometrial thickness; INR and FBC	May need hysteroscopy/ D&C as day case/inpatient
3. Secondary infertility	Mid-luteal progesterone, day-2 FSH, USS pelvis, sperm count; will need HSG	Routine gynaecology clinic/ fertility clinic
4. DUB in obese pt	FBC, HbA1C. USS pelvis, pregnancy test	Urgent appt in view of obesity and attendant risks; will need hysteroscopy/ D&C
5. Pelvic mass, nulliparous	FBC, Ca 125, USS pelvis	General gynae clinic; urgent as nature of pelvic mass not yet confirmed
6. Prolapse with urinary symptoms	MSU	Routine, ideally pelvic floor clinic or someone who has an interest in urogynae
7. Possible cervical polyp or ectropion	Check smear result	Options, general gynae or colposcopy clinic; wait time depends on the smear result; may need cryo or cautery (see & treat)
8. Pelvic pain, possibly infertility, likely to be endometriosis	USS pelvis, FBC and ESR	Routine gynaecology, likely to need diagnostic laparoscopy at the least
9. Pruritus vulvae, need to establish a diagnosis	Urine dipstick; may need HbA1C and possible biopsy of the area	Need to exclude vulval dermatosis; may need dermovate and emollients
10. Raised prolactin, will need imaging to exclude microadenoma, FSH/LH may be due to OCP	Pregnancy and thyroid function tests	Ideally reproductive medicine; routine; may need optical fundoscopy

Mark sheet

Letter 1

0   1   2   3   4

Letter 2

0   1   2   3   4

Letter 3

0   1   2   3   4

Letter 4

0   1   2   3   4

Letter 5

0   1   2   3   4

Letter 6

0   1   2   3   4

Letter 7

0   1   2   3   4

Letter 8

0   1   2   3   4

Letter 9

0   1   2   3   4

Letter 10

0   1   2   3   4

Divide scores by 2:

Total: /20

Operative – Caesarean section

Candidate's instructions

You are the registrar coming on duty at the time of routine handover. Mrs Jones is in Room 6. She is a primip at term who has been in labour for over 14 hours. She has had an effective epidural sited and, despite the use of syntocinon, her cervix has remained at 9 cm dilatation over the last 2–3 hours.

On abdominal examination, there is one-fifth of the head palpable, confirmed on bimanual examination with caput and moulding of the head. The CTG has remained normal throughout, despite a trace of meconium on her pad. A decision has already been made for the patient to have a CS and you will have to do it.

You have 14 minutes during which the examiner will ask you seven questions. You will be asked by the examiner to describe in detail:

- the steps required in relation to the decision for LSCS, discussion, consent preparation
- the procedure itself
- the patient's postoperative care and the plan for future pregnancies.

Examiner's instructions and mark sheet

You need to ask the candidate to describe in detail the steps required in relation to the decision for lower-segment CS (LSCS), discussion, consent preparation and the procedure itself, the patient's postoperative care, and the plan for future pregnancies. Seven questions appear on the mark sheet.

You will cover aspects of the procedure that relate to CS in general, as well as the factors that relate to this specific case.

1. Comment on the decision to perform the CS.

- Appropriate decision
- Most likely OP/OT position
- With some head palpable abdominally, then vaginal delivery would be inappropriate

0   1   2

2. What preoperative measures need to be undertaken?

- Consent
- Group & save if not already done
- Antacids
- Urinary catheter
- Thromboprophylaxis may need to be reassessed (should have been done at the booking visit)

0   1   2   3

3. What type of anaesthesia would be appropriate?

- Top-up epidural or, if thought inadequate, then spinal
- GA may be necessary but ideally use regional block

0   1   2

4. What is the degree of urgency for this CS?

- Within 30 minutes as the CTG has been normal

0   1

5. Take me through the procedure and what you would expect to find.

- May need a shave
- Prepare the skin with iodine solution or other antiseptic
- Describe opening the abdomen
- Expectation of free fluid in the abdomen
- Oedematous lower segment
- Transverse incision across lower segment
- Likely to be OP/OT position, head may need flexing and rotating, may be able to deliver manually, may need forceps
- Cord pH
- Deliver placenta and check cavity empty
- Patient given syntocinon and antibiotics intravenously with delivery of the baby (as risk of primary postpartum haemorrhage (PPH), consider an intravenous infusion to avoid poor contractility of the uterus)
- Describe closure of lower segment
- Check ovaries/tubes and that bleeding settled
- Describe routine closure of the abdomen
- May swab out the vagina
- Ensure appropriate operation notes and intraoperative findings

0   1   2   3   4   5   6   7

6. What would be your instructions for her postoperative care?

- Leave catheter until mobile
- Check thromboprophylaxis is written up
- May continue antibiotics for 24 hours
- Adequate analgesia
- Fluids and diet as tolerated
- Early mobilization
- Will need to check FBC before discharge

0   1   2   3

7. Are there any other concerns you would have for this patient?

- She has been adequately debriefed
- She could not have done anything differently
- Brief discussion about future pregnancies and decision about vaginal birth after CS (VBAC)

0   1   2

Total: /20

Abnormal smear

Candidate's instructions

The patient's GP has referred the woman you are about to see to your colposcopy clinic. A copy of the referral letter is given below. You have 14 minutes to read the letter and obtain a relevant history from the patient. You should discuss any relevant investigations and treatment that you feel may be indicated.

The Surgery
High Road
Buckhurst Hill

Dear Doctor

Re: Mrs Joan Starr, aged 30 years

I would be pleased if you could see this patient whose recent cervical smear result showed moderate dyskaryosis with wart viral infection. She is nulliparous and the rest of her medical history is unremarkable.

Yours sincerely

Dr S White

Marks will be awarded for:

- relevant history-taking
- discussion of relevant investigations
- discussion of relevant treatment options.

Role-player's brief

- You are Joan Starr, a 30-year-old woman who works as a secretary. You have been completely freaked out by this result and have two things on your mind:
  - you think this result means that you have got cancer
  - your husband has been unfaithful and has given you the wart virus, and this is entirely his fault.
- You are completely asymptomatic.
- You have never been pregnant and have never had any sexually transmitted diseases. You have only ever had three sexual partners and do not really like talking about sexual matters.
- You are taking the pill but no other medication and have no other medical history of note.
- You smoke 20 cigarettes a day but this has recently increased since discovering the smear result.
- Your mother died from breast cancer at the age of 54 years and you are worried that her history and your abnormal smear result may be linked.
- You are anxious to know more about the procedure of colposcopy: will it hurt and how long will it take for the results? You want to know the treatment options and might consider alternative therapies because you are afraid of hospitals.
- You are also anxious about your fertility as you were planning to stop the pill to try for a pregnancy and only had the smear taken to check all was well before doing so. This is your first smear as you have previously avoided having them performed.

Examiner's instructions and mark sheet

Familiarize yourself with the candidate's instructions. At this station the candidate will have 14 minutes to obtain a history relevant to the patient's complaint. The candidate should also discuss with the patient what a colposcopy entails and that a biopsy may be necessary. Do not award half marks.

The candidate needs to explain to the patient that cytology is looking for a premalignant lesion, and to sensibly explain what the term 'wart virus infection' means.

History

- Checks the patient's age and date of her LMP
- Menstrual history – any bleeding between the periods or after intercourse (IMB/PCB)
- Basic gynaecological history/contraception/fertility issues
- Obstetric history
- Genital tract infections
- Family and social history, including smoking
- Medical history
- Allergies, especially to iodine

0   1   2   3   4   5   6

Colposcopy counselling

- The smear suggests a premalignant (precancer) lesion
- Explain what happens: positioning her legs in stirrups, uses acetic acid and iodine on the cervix, procedure usually takes 5–10 minutes
- Biopsy is usually needed
- Colposcopy usually gives an impression of the underlying cause for the abnormal smear
- Explain that the NHS cervical screening programme (CSP) is screening for premalignant disease and the incidence of cervical cancer in the UK is 2000–3000 new cases per year
- More than likely needs treatment
- Avoid blaming any particular partner

0   1   2   3   4   5   6

Treatment

- Advise stopping smoking and explain that smoking affects the local immunity on the cervix
- Explain about loop excision of the transformation zone (LLETZ) and that it could be done as an outpatient under local anaesthetic or as a day case under general anaesthetic (GA)
- Could see and treat today but if she is anxious then may be better to get a diagnosis first
- Target times associated with the NHS CSP and consequently will not have a long wait
- Will need follow-up after treatment (1 in 20 may need a further treatment)
- At some point, explain that this should not affect her fertility (i.e. getting pregnant) though may increase her risk of going into labour prematurely.

0   1   2   3   4   5   6

Role-player's score

0   1   2

(2 = role-player happy to see candidate again, 1 = prepared to see candidate again, 0 = never wants to see candidate again).

Total: /20

CTG abnormality

Candidate's instructions

You are called to see Mrs Dunne in Room 4. She is a 28-year-old primip who is now 7 days past her due date (EDD) in an otherwise uneventful first pregnancy. She was booked for induction of labour in 4 days' time. She has presented with some irregular contractions, decreased fetal movements and a mucoid discharge ('show'). The midwife is worried about the CTG which she shows you.

You have 14 minutes to counsel the patient about the management of the labour. Her vital signs are normal. The presentation of the fetus is cephalic and the head is engaged. The midwife performed a VE and found the cervix to be 1–2 cm dilated but fully effaced and the head was 2 cm above the ischial spines.

Marks will be awarded for:

- discussing the CTG
- discussing further management of this labour.

Role-player's brief

- You are Sarah Dunne, 28 years old, and you live with your partner who works for Everychild (a non-governmental organization, NGO).
- Your pregnancy has been lovely and you feel very well in yourself. Your midwife has been absolutely wonderful.
- You had initially wanted a home birth with as little intervention as possible, but your midwife persuaded you that this might not be best for the baby as this was your first one.
- You have been well throughout the pregnancy and all the scans and blood tests have been normal. You noticed some tightenings during the night with a show and slight decrease in the baby's movements. You are convinced it is a girl and keep calling her Flora.
- Your partner is devoted to you and is on his way from work. You are reluctant to be monitored and do so grudgingly for Flora's sake, but feel that the whole of the medical profession is male-dominated and wants to do CSs on everyone.
- You are concerned about the welfare of your baby and want the registrar to be very explicit about why he is worried about the trace. If he does not pick up on the severity of the trace, you need to get him to explain why it doesn't look like the one in your book by Miriam Stoppard.

Examiner's instructions

Familiarize yourself with the candidate's instructions. The candidate is asked to:

- discuss the CTG
- discuss a further management plan for her labour.

Score the candidate's performance on the mark sheet. The role player will have a maximum of 2 marks to award the candidate. You should not interact with the candidate.

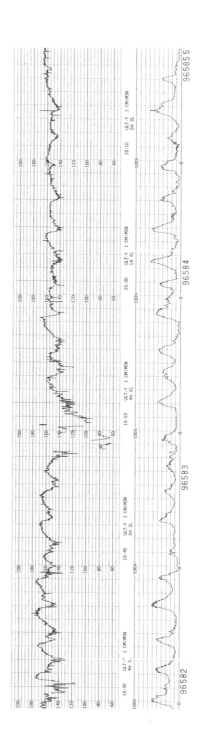

Mark sheet

Do not award half marks.

Discussion of CTG under broad headings

- Define risk, decreased fetal movements and past due date
- Contraction regularity
- Baseline rate – tachycardia
- Variability – reduced
- Accelerations – none
- Decelerations – shallow
- Opinion – the CTG is not reassuring/abnormal, showing a complicated tachycardia, and this is very worrying at such an early stage of labour

0   1   2   3   4   5   6

Concern about status of the fetus

- Early stage of labour as she is only 1–2 cm and may be in labour for another 8 hours (cervical dilatation at 1 cm per hour)
- The fetus is already showing signs of distress on the CTG, may have passed meconium, so it may be worth rupturing her membranes
- Will need to maintain the CTG for the time being
- Unable to do FBS as only 1–2 cm and, if doing an FBS at this stage, may have to be repeated numerous times
- Possible diagnosis could be abruption or feto-maternal transfusion

0   1   2   3   4

Concern about status of the mother

- Need to continue monitoring the mother (pulse, BP and temperature) as well as input and output.
- Suggest FBC, U&Es, clotting if abruption considered, as well as group & save
- Needs intravenous access

0   1   2   3

Discussion of LSCS

- Type of anaesthesia (spinal versus GA), allows partner to be present if patient awake

- Consent form needs to be signed
- Portrays the urgency of the situation
- Paediatricians will be asked to be present
- Possibility that the baby may have to go to the neonatal unit
- Will allow skin-to-skin contact depending on condition of the baby

0   1   2   3   4   5

Role-player's score

0   1   2

(2 = role-player happy to see candidate again, 1 = prepared to see candidate again, 0 = never wants to see candidate again).

Total: /20

CIRCUIT B, STATION 8

Interactive viva

Candidate's instructions

> **THIS IS A FIVE-PART STATION.**

It follows the course of a pregnancy in a grand multip. At each stage, you will be asked a question about the scenario.

Once you have dealt with each part of the question, you should progress to the next part. You cannot go back to a section once finished. You have 14 minutes.

PART A

Mrs AK is a 40-year-old woman of Asian origin. She has a history of regular periods. She presents to the antenatal clinic for booking at 24 weeks' gestation, having just come back from Pakistan. She is gravida 10, para 7 + 3 miscarriages. She has had seven full-term normal deliveries over the past 15 years; her youngest child is 4 years old. There were no apparent problems with any of the pregnancies. The weights of the babies were each normal for their gestational ages.

Despite having had all her children in the UK, her English is limited.

Mrs AK has recently been diagnosed as having non-insulin dependent diabetes. There is a family history of hypertension.

Her BMI is 29.4. Her blood pressure was initially recorded at 138/91 mmHg, but this appeared to settle to 120/70 using a large cuff. On dipstick testing of her urine there were 1+ proteinuria. The detailed scan which was performed just prior to clinic was normal and confirmed her gestational age.

> **DISCUSS YOUR MANAGEMENT PLAN FOR THIS PATIENT'S PREGNANCY.**

PART B

Mrs AK attends the antenatal clinic at 31 weeks' gestation. Her blood sugars are not well controlled and her weight has increased by 8 kg. She is still using metformin and measuring her BMs pre- and post-prandially. Her blood pressure is becoming problematic at 140/100 mmHg, even using a large cuff. She feels well in herself and the fetal movements are normal.

On examination in the clinic, her BP is persistently 150/100. Her reflexes were normal and there was no clonus. The fundal height was equivalent to dates and the fetal heart was present. Her urine showed 3+ proteinuria on testing.

> **DISCUSS YOUR PLAN OF MANAGEMENT AT THIS STAGE.**

PART C

Mrs AK is admitted to the ward from clinic, at 31 weeks' gestation. She is converted to insulin and her blood sugars come under control quite quickly and she becomes confident about injecting herself.

However her blood pressure is a little more difficult to control. After 48 hours there is some discussion about whether delivery should be expedited.

The growth of the baby appears normal and all the mother's blood tests are normal and stable.

On your morning ward round, her husband is present who speaks good English. Mrs AK is concerned about what might happen if the baby needed to be delivered now.

> **WHAT INFORMATION SHOULD YOU PROVIDE TO THE PARENTS ABOUT THE PROBLEMS THE BABY MAY ENCOUNTER IF DELIVERED AT THIS GESTATION?**

PART D

Mrs AK's blood pressure and blood sugars have stabilized. She is now 36 weeks pregnant and all seems to be going well. The growth of the baby seems to be satisfactory but the lie is unstable and currently is presenting as a breech presentation.

> **WHAT WOULD BE YOUR ONGOING MANAGEMENT OF THIS PATIENT?**

PART E

Mrs AK presents to the labour ward at 37 weeks' gestation with a history of regular contractions and spontaneous rupture of membranes. The presentation is cephalic and appears to be fixed in the pelvis. The cervix is 3 cm dilated with the head at station –2 cm. Her blood pressure is 140/100 mmHg, but she has no obvious symptoms.

HOW WOULD YOU MANAGE HER LABOUR?

Examiner's instructions and mark sheet

Please read the candidate's instructions. Ask the questions as they appear on the sheet and do not prompt. The scoring should be awarded globally.

PART A

Question: Discuss your management plan for this patient's pregnancy

- Immediate – check FBC, sickle and U&Es as baselines
- Regular blood sugar monitoring, and refer to diabetes team for assessment to decide whether she needs to go on insulin
- MSU and possible 24-hour urine for protein
- Make an appropriate plan for getting her BP checked
- Arrange regular ultrasound scans for growth of the fetus
- Will need active third stage

0   1   2   3   4

PART B

Question: Discuss your plan of management at this stage

- The mother
  - Commence antihypertensive – labetalol
  - Probably needs starting on insulin
  - As English limited, may need to consider admission to stabilize her BP and blood sugars
  - Check bloods including FBC, U&Es, urate and liver function tests (LFTs)
  - MSU and consider commencing a 24-hour urine
- The fetus
  - CTG
  - USS to check growth and estimate of weight

0   1   2   3   4

PART C

Question: What information should you provide to the parents about the problems the baby may encounter if delivered at this gestation?

- Emphasize that the baby is 9 weeks early
- Outlook at this gestation good especially as the baby is normally grown
- Breathing problems may occur and may need ventilation

- Mother might benefit from a course of steroids and, if so, would need to go on a sliding scale as blood sugars may be affected
- Feeding may produce some difficulties, and so may need to be fed by nasogastric (NG) tube
- May need to be in an incubator for temperature control
- Will probably need to stay in hospital until the due date
- Babies at this gestation can have problems with jaundice

0   1   2   3   4

PART D

Question: What would be your ongoing management of this patient?

- Routine bloods for 36 weeks
- Weekly or bi-weekly BP monitoring
- Continue blood sugar monitoring
- Consider external cephatic version (ECV) at 36–38 weeks and possible stabilizing induction
- Elective CS at 38 weeks may be an option and offer sterilization
- Ensure VTE assessment has been done, as she booked late

0   1   2   3   4

PART E

Question: How would you manage her labour?

- The mother
  - Regular monitoring of BP
  - Check reflexes and the presence of clonus
  - Check FBC, U&Es, LFTs
  - Input and output chart
  - Sliding scale of insulin
  - May want to consider epidural or other form of analgesia
  - If BP rises then may need to be placed on the appropriate labour ward protocol
  - Active management of the labour
- The fetus
  - Continuous CTG monitoring
  - Need active third stage of labour
  - May want to inform paediatricians

0   1   2   3   4

Total: /20

Ectopic pregnancy – explain laparoscopy

Candidate's instructions

The casualty officer initially referred the patient you are about to see. You have already seen Veronica Morgan (who is a Jehovah's Witness (JW)) in the Accident and Emergency (A&E) department with a history of vaginal spotting and severe right iliac fossa pain, which had been present for 6 hours. She is otherwise fit and well. The only medical history of note is that she had her appendix removed when she was 10 years old. She has been trying to conceive over the past 18 months and her LMP was 7 weeks ago. She was thrilled when her pregnancy test was positive.

On your original assessment you suspected an ectopic pregnancy. As her observations were stable you asked for an urgent ultrasound scan. The scan shows an empty uterus, a 2 cm adnexal swelling on the right side and some fluid in the Pouch of Douglas (presumably blood).

You feel she needs a laparoscopy. You have 14 minutes to explain the suspected diagnosis to Ms Morgan and the proposed management.

Marks will be awarded for:

- explaining the diagnosis
- discussing treatment options
- identifying and answering the patient's concerns.

Role-player's brief

- You are Veronica Morgan, a 28-year-old woman who works as a personal assistant. You have been trying to become pregnant over the past 18 months.
- You have presented with some vaginal bleeding and quite severe pain in the right lower quadrant of your abdomen. You have already done a home pregnancy test, which was positive.
- You have had a vaginal scan, which was uncomfortable, and are waiting for the registrar to talk to you about the results.
- He is going to tell you that the pregnancy is in the tube and that you will need a laparoscopy (telescope) into the abdomen and may need some other form of surgery. You have no idea about your reproductive anatomy and must get him to explain in non-technical terms.
- As he continues to explain, you realize that you have lost the pregnancy whatever happens, and you get very emotional about that. You are also worried about future fertility and contraception.
- You are a Jehovah's Witness and are adamant about no blood products.

Prompt for questions

- 'Why is it not in the womb?'
- 'Can't it be moved into the womb?'
- 'Can I go and see my GP to discuss it?'
- 'I need to talk to my husband'
- 'Are there any drugs that can be used to salvage the pregnancy?'
- Ask about future fertility, as you have been trying for 18 months to get pregnant.
- 'What are the risks of it happening again?'
- 'I don't want a hysterectomy'
- 'Are you going to kill my baby and what is going to happen to it?'
- 'Are you telling me I am going to have an abortion?'

Examiner's instructions and mark sheet

General – explaining the diagnosis

- Explain the diagnosis of tubal pregnancy correctly (ideally with a diagram); i.e. 7 weeks of amenorrhoea, positive pregnancy test and an empty uterus on ultrasound scan
- One would expect to see a fetal heart in the uterine cavity by this stage
- This is a non-viable pregnancy
- Acknowledge pregnancy loss/bereavement aspect
- Need to intervene as she has signs of peritonism
- Risk of rupture if it hasn't already

0   1   2   3   4   5

Treatment

- Explain proposed management laparoscopy (possible laparotomy)
- Explain the procedure of the above, how it is done
- Will need a GA
- Explain differences in salpingostomy/salpingectomy (RCOG guidelines)
- May have adhesions from previous appendix and that may need division and may have been a predisposing factor in this case
- Aim to undertake laparoscopically – will need thromboembolic deterrent (TED) stockings

0   1   2   3   4   5

Discussion of future fertility

- Ovarian function will be unchanged, aim to conserve the ovaries
- Risk of a further ectopic (1 in 8 chance)
- Discuss future types of contraception to avoid (progestogens)

0   1   2   3   4

Dealing with JW aspect

- Talk about the possibility of large blood loss
- Need to test for blood group and risk of isoimmunization
- Possible autotransfusion
- Discuss patient signing a separate consent form
- Recognize patient's autonomy

0   1   2   3   4

Role-player's score

0   1   2

(2 = role-player happy to see candidate again, 1 = prepared to see candidate again, 0 = never wants to see candidate again).

Total: /20

CIRCUIT B, STATION 10

Breech delivery

Candidate's instructions

Delivery unit emergency call

Doctor, please come to Room 6 immediately, Mrs Grayson gravida 4, para 3, under the care of an independent midwife, is in advanced labour with an undiagnosed breech presentation.

You have 14 minutes during which you are asked to discuss with the examiner how you would proceed and will then be asked a number of questions pertinent to the case. A doll and mannequin are available for you to take the examiner through a breech delivery.

You will be awarded marks for:

- dealing appropriately with the situation
- conduct of the breech delivery
- answering satisfactorily the examiner's subsequent questions.

Examiner's instructions and mark sheet

Question for the candidate

'Take me through what you would do.'

Prompt

'Would you like any other information?'

Information available

- Patient aged 35 years
- Normal pregnancy
- Normal obstetric history
  - SVD: 3.4 kg
  - SVD: 3.6 kg
  - SVD: 3.6 kg
  - all term babies
- Term for this pregnancy
- SRM, 2 hours previously, no meconium
- Observations normal, fetal HR 150 bpm, intermittent auscultation
- VE fully dilated
- Breech RSL distending introitus with contractions
- Doll and pelvis present for the candidate to take examiner through breech delivery

Once the candidate has finished the delivery, the following questions should be asked:

- 'What is the role of ECV in this case?'
- 'What are the contraindications to ECV?'
- 'How would you have managed this patient had you seen her the week prior to delivery?'

Mark sheet

Asking about appropriate history

- Age and gestation of the patient
- Any antenatal problems
- Previous obstetric history, courses of the labours and weights of the babies
- Are the membranes intact
- Colour of the liquor
- Cervical dilatation and station of the presenting part
- Type of breech, any cord palpable
- Any problems with the fetal heart
- Any problems with the patient's vital signs

0   1   2   3   4   5

Examining the patient

- Check the size of the baby
- Presenting part and its level of descent
- Check vaginal findings and may ask to empty the patient's bladder

0   1   2

Conduct of breech delivery

- Places mannequin in lithotomy, brings the buttocks to the end of the bed/table
- Allows the breech to distend the perineum with contractions and maternal effort
- Considers episiotomy
- Avoids touching the presenting part if possible
- May place fingers on the sacrum and bony pelvis to guide the rotation of the baby
- Keeps baby's sacrum and back anterior (uppermost) and may need to hold the baby to avoid counter rotation
- If extended breech, flexes the knee to deliver them
- May need to help deliver arms by flexing over the baby's chest
- Allows the baby to hang
- Asks for assistance, draws the legs upwards with a cloth around the legs, avoiding touching the abdomen.

- Delivery of aftercoming head with either forceps, or Mauriceau Smellie Veit manoeuvre (avoids pulling on the jaw and understands the importance of keeping the head flexed with malar pressure)

0   1   2   3   4   5   6   7   8

Answers the examiner's questions appropriately

- ECV has no role in this case
- Contraindications to ECV
  - ante partum haemorrhage (APH) in this pregnancy
  - Ruptured membranes
  - Multiple pregnancy
  - Severe fetal abnormality
  - If CS needed for another indication
  - IUGR
  - Severe PET/hypertension
  - Uterine abnormality
  - Cord around the neck
  - Abnormal CTG
- Managed her the previous week
  - Offer her ECV, possibly a stabilizing induction
  - Offer her an elective LSCS

0   1   2   3   4   5

Total: /20

Medical ethics and the law – preparatory station

Candidate's instructions

This is a preparatory station and you have 15 minutes to read through the four case scenarios, which present ethical and medico-legal problems. You will then meet the examiner to discuss all the cases over the course of 14 minutes.

In each case you need to identify the main ethical and/or medico-legal issue and suggest how each situation can best be managed.

Marks will be awarded for:

- identifying the underlying ethical and/or medico-legal issue
- suggesting how you feel each situation should be managed.

CASE 1

An experienced family planning doctor saw Kate Braithwaite in the family planning clinic a few weeks ago. Kate is 15 years old and was requesting the oral contraceptive pill (OCP) as her relationship with her boyfriend had become sexually intimate and she wanted to ensure that she did not become pregnant.

The doctor discussed safe sex and barrier methods but at the end of the consultation felt that Kate was acting responsibly and consequently prescribed her the combined OCP. She did, however, suggest that Kate discuss this with her parents, or at least with her mother.

Two weeks later, her mother was tidying in her daughter's bedroom when she came across the packet of OCPs and confronted her daughter. She has turned up to the clinic demanding to see the doctor who prescribed the OCP to her 'under-age' daughter and questioning the morality of the doctor concerned. She also questioned why she or her husband, who is a vicar, were not consulted and questioned the legality of the situation.

CASE 2

Imelda Volgin is a 26-year-old woman in her second pregnancy. She booked late in this pregnancy as she had recently been back home to eastern Europe. She is now 22 weeks pregnant and all her blood tests are normal.

However, her detailed ultrasound scan has shown that her baby has Potter's syndrome (absent kidneys), which is incompatible with extrauterine life. She has been seen by the fetal medicine team who have confirmed the diagnosis. She is very shocked by the findings and feels unable to make a decision about terminating the pregnancy until she has discussed it with her husband and family. She is not totally against a termination but doesn't want to regret her decision.

CASE 3

Mrs Patsy Gerrard is a 46-year-old Afro-Caribbean woman from Trinidad. She has been referred to the gynaecology clinic with a history of heavy, painful periods and some intermenstrual bleeding. A recent Hb was 8.5 g/dL with a low mean corpuscular volume (MCV), suggesting an iron-deficiency anaemia.

Clinically, she appears pale and has a fibroid uterus up to the level of her umbilicus. She has had a recent hysteroscopy and endometrial sampling, which did not show any endometrial abnormality.

A long discussion was undertaken in the clinic. It was obvious that she needs a hysterectomy to resolve her problems. However, she mentioned that she is a Jehovah's Witness and is adamant that she will not have a blood transfusion under any circumstances.

CASE 4

Joan Bryce is a 48-year-old woman with a history of large uterine fibroids causing pressure symptoms. The size of the uterus is equivalent to 28 weeks' gestation.

She has had an MRI scan and been discussed at the local multidisciplinary team (MDT) meeting to exclude any possibility of malignancy within the fibroids. Her most recent blood count was normal.

After discussion it has been decided that her best option would be a total abdominal hysterectomy. She has decided that she would like to have her ovaries conserved unless there is bleeding at the time of the operation that can only be stopped by their removal.

Everything seems straightforward, until the consultant is informed by her husband that she was diagnosed with pre-senile dementia 2 years ago. The surgery is planned for the following week.

Examiner's instructions

Familiarize yourself with the candidate's instructions and the case summaries.

The candidate is asked to discuss with you:

- the underlying ethical and/or medico-legal issue for each case
- a management plan or logical approach to each case.

You should avoid prompting the candidate, but ask the following questions for each case:

- 'What do you think are the underlying ethical and/or medico-legal issues in this case?'
- 'What would be your suggested management approach in each case?'

Mark sheet

Each station is marked out of 5. Do not award half marks.

CASE 1

Issues

- Confidentiality – duty of care of the doctor is to the patient and not a relative, and the Data Protection Act (1998) does not allow disclosure of patient information to a third party.
- Gillick competency/Fraser guidelines (1985) ruling that it is not illegal to prescribe contraception to under-16s provided they understand the consequences and risks.

Dealing with the issues

- Advise the mother that the case can be discussed only in general terms, quoting the guidelines and the Data Protection Act.
- The doctor should not discuss the individual case as it is a breach of confidentiality and the girl would have been told that her confidentiality would be respected.
- Could offer to meet with the parents and the girl if the daughter agrees.
- The mother may want to consider the risk of termination of pregnancy.
- There has been no illegality in dealing with this case.

0   1   2   3   4   5

CASE 2

Issues

- Termination of pregnancy is covered in the Abortion Act (1991) and, under clause E, is permissible at any stage of the pregnancy if the fetal condition is incompatible with life. Ideally, one would recommend termination as early as possible.

Dealing with the issues

- Patient needs to be satisfied that termination is the correct course of action for her.
- If she decides on a termination then she will need mefipristone followed by cervagem, or follow the local protocol.
- If she decides against termination, then routine antenatal care.
- If she decides on a termination later than 22 weeks, then it may be appropriate to undertake feticide prior to delivery.

- Would need follow-up and be offered bereavement counselling.
- Post-mortem and chromosome analysis should be offered.

0   1   2   3   4   5

CASE 3
Issues

- Patient autonomy needs to be respected. It would be considered assault to give a blood transfusion to a Jehovah's Witness against their wishes and may run the risk of being reported to the General Medical Council (GMC) as well as being taken to court.

Dealing with the issues

- Attempt to stop her menstrual periods with either high-dose progestogens or GnRH analogues.
- Commence oral iron and optimize her haemoglobin.
- Separate consent form, and patient may seek JW advocate.
- Discuss the possibility of autologous transfusion depending on her wishes.
- Cell saver should be used in theatre.

0   1   2   3   4   5

CASE 4
Issues

- Patient's capacity to consent needs to be assessed; this is governed by the Mental Capacity Act 2005.

Dealing with the issues

- The four tests of capacity are to assess the patient's:
  - Understanding of the information given
  - Ability to retain that information
  - Ability to decide on an issue
  - Ability to communicate her understanding of the procedure.
- Treatment can proceed without consent if it is in the patient's best interests.
- No-one else can give consent, but relatives or unpaid carers should be involved in the discussions.
- In some cases the patient may need an independent advocate, a second opinion and hospital legal adviser.
- A court order is only rarely necessary for contentious treatments.

0   1   2   3   4   5

Total: /20

Shoulder dystocia – teaching station

Candidate's instructions

You have been asked by the department's tutor to teach the fourth-year medical student attached to your firm about shoulder dystocia following a case the student saw yesterday. This is the student's first week of obstetrics and gynaecology (O&G) and he/she was disturbed by the event. The tutor feels that having a one-to-one with the student may allay his/her anxieties.

A doll and mannequin have been provided to help you demonstrate this obstetric emergency. You have 14 minutes at this station.

You will be marked on your ability to:

- explain the significance of shoulder dystocia
- teach the medical student (role-player) how to deal with it.

Role-player's brief

- You are Emma Bond, a fourth-year medical student and have been doing your first undergraduate time in O&G.
- You spent some time on the labour ward last night and the woman who you were observing had a shoulder dystocia. You found the whole procedure distressing. You explained this to the tutor and it has been arranged that one of the registrars will teach you today about shoulder dystocia.
- The candidate is supposed to talk to you about the significance of shoulder dystocia. If he or she doesn't cover the following points, then you should ask:
  - 'What are the predisposing factors to shoulder dystocia?'
  - 'How often does it occur in normal-weight babies?'
  - 'How quickly does the cord pH fall?'

Examiner's instructions and mark sheet

Familiarize yourself with the candidate's instructions. The candidate is asked to:

- explain the significance of shoulder dystocia
- teach the medical student (role-player) how to deal with a shoulder dystocia.

Score the candidate's performance on the mark sheet. The role player will have a maximum of 2 marks to award the candidate. You should not interact with the candidate. Do not award half marks.

Setting the scene

- It is an emergency situation that is usually covered in the 'drills and skills' tutorials.
- It occurs in babies of normal weight in 50 per cent of cases.
- Predisposing factors include gestational diabetes mellitus (GDM), raised body mass index (BMI) of mother, large baby, post-maturity.
- The urgency relates to the fall in cord pH which drops at 0.04/minute. How well a baby fares depends on the timing, especially if the baby is already compromised.
- Candidate explains how he or she plans to demonstrate the manoeuvres, allows the role-player to demonstrate them by assisting and then observing.

| 0 | 1 | 2 | 3 | 4 |

(adjust mark if role-player has to prompt)

Manoeuvres in delivery of the shoulders

H Call for help: anaesthetist, paediatrician and labour ward coordinator.

E Evaluate for episiotomy. If she hasn't had an episiotomy, it may be worth performing one.

L Legs – place in McRobert's position. That is hyperflexed at the hips and flexed at the knee. Usually the baby delivers at this stage. If not, then proceed to:

P Pressure – continuous or intermittent (rocking) suprapubic external pressure behind the anterior shoulder, understanding of the direction of pressure, identifying which way the head is facing anteriorly.

E Enter vagina with fingers.
  - Rubin manoeuvre: approach anterior fetal shoulder from its posterior aspect in order to adduct the shoulder; i.e. reduce the biacromial diameters and rotate to the oblique.

- Woods screw manoeuvre: approach the posterior fetal shoulder from its anterior aspect and gently rotate towards the symphysis.
- Reverse Woods screw manoeuvre: approach the posterior shoulder from its posterior aspect and attempt to dislodge in the opposite direction to the above.

R Remove the arm. Follow the posterior arm down to the elbow and flex the arm at the elbow and sweep the forearm across the chest.

R Roll the patient over on to all fours as it increases the pelvic diameters. Movement and gravity may aid in dislodging the impacted shoulder and aim to deliver the posterior shoulder.

Continue each for 30 seconds before moving on to the manoeuvre. Ensure someone is keeping watch on the time and shouting out after each 30 seconds.

0   1   2   3   4   5   6   7   8

Demonstrates the procedure adequately

0   1   2

Takes the role-player through the procedure

0   1   2

Allows role-player to demonstrate what he/she has been taught

0   1   2

Role-player's score

0   1   2

(0 = no confidence in being able to deal with shoulder dystocia, 1= reasonably confident, fully confident).

Total: /20

CIRCUIT C, STATION 3

Ovarian cyst

Candidate's instructions

The next patient you will see is Mrs Dunlop who is 45 years old and has been referred to your clinic by her GP.

She had a recent admission under the general surgeons with abdominal pain, which settled overnight with analgesia. She had then discharged herself before any further investigations could be performed. An enthusiastic FY2 had sent off a battery of tests including a Ca125 during her recent admission as she was found to have a swelling in the pelvis on rectal examination.

She went to see her GP and, on closer questioning, appeared also to have had some menstrual problems.

At the time of the latest referral a full blood count (FBC) as well as an ultrasound scan of her abdomen and pelvis were requested. This has been performed just prior to coming to clinic and the result she brings shows there is a complex mass 8 cm in diameter in the pelvis consistent with a lesion arising from the left ovary. The mass is partly solid and partly cystic with some free fluid in the Pouch of Douglas (POD). The right ovary and uterus are normal. The liver appears normal and there is no other abnormality of note. The FBC shows a haemoglobin of 10.8 g/dL and the Ca125 level is 65.

You have 14 minutes to take a relevant history, explain the possible differential diagnosis and discuss her ongoing management.

Marks will be awarded for:

- taking a relevant history
- explaining the scan findings
- discussing the differential diagnoses
- discussing her ongoing management.

Role-player's brief

- You are Gillian Dunlop, a 45-year-old housewife with two children aged 12 and 14 years.
- You have been feeling run-down but felt that it was due to some sleepless nights with your 14-year-old. You had a recent hospital admission when you had acute lower abdominal pain which settled overnight, and you discharged yourself because you were worried about your children but also because you do not like hospitals.
- On questioning you give a history of heavy periods during which you lose clots and have associated pain. You also have been getting pain with intercourse which appears to be getting worse.
- You have had two full-term normal deliveries.
- Your last cervical smear test was taken 6 months ago and was normal, but it was painful when the speculum was inserted.
- You are a non-smoker. You have no other medical history of note. You do not take any medication and have no allergies.
- Your husband had a vasectomy in the past.
- You initially thought you might have an ulcer. The radiographer said you had an ovarian cyst and it would all be explained in clinic. The diagnosis as far as you are concerned is that of an ovarian cyst and you want to know what the doctor would recommend.
- If the candidate mentions cancer, then ask if he or she is sure of the diagnosis. You knew someone who had ovarian cancer, who died very quickly after being told of the diagnosis, and you are worried about your children.

Examiner's instructions and mark sheet

Familiarize yourself with the candidate's instructions. The candidate is asked to:

- take a relevant history
- explain the scan findings
- discuss the differential diagnoses
- discuss the patient's ongoing management.

Score the candidate's performance on the mark sheet. The role-player will have a maximum of 2 marks to award the candidate. You should not interact with the candidate. Do not award half marks.

Taking a relevant history

- Pain – its nature and features
- Menstrual history
- History of dysmenorrhea and dyspareunia
- Obstetric history
- Fertility issues/contraception
- Genital tract infections
- Bowel problems
- Appetite and weight loss
- Urinary symptoms
- Family history

0   1   2   3   4   5

Explaining the scan findings

- Sensitive manner in explaining nature of the cyst in light of Ca125 level
- Ca125 level raised which is very sensitive but not specific
- Relative malignant index (RMI) <200

0   1   2   3

Discussion of differential diagnosis

- Endometriosis
- Possible torsion of the cyst (cause of her visit to Accident and Emergency (A&E))
- Pelvic inflammatory disease (PID)
- Hydro- or haemato-salpinx
- Fibroid

- Cancer, primary/secondary
- Tuberculosis

0   1   2   3   4

Discussion of ongoing management

- In view of size of cyst, it will need surgery at some stage
- RMI <200
- May be worth repeating the Ca125
- MRI scan with contrast to delineate the anatomy
- May need a CT scan if hint of malignancy (protocols may vary between cancer networks)
- Aspiration of fluid for cytology under ultrasound may be necessary depending on MDT review
- In view of raised Ca125, get the investigations as 'Target' so expediting results
- MDT review images to decide on what is the most appropriate surgery:
  - If benign then just oophorectomy/cystectomy
  - If endometriosis then laparoscopic surgery may be appropriate
  - If malignant then more radical surgery
- Cancer target – explain about the timely nature of these targets
- Check routine blood tests and other tumour markers

0   1   2   3   4   5   6

Role-player's score

0   1   2

(2 = role-player happy to see candidate again, 1 = prepared to see candidate again, 0 = never wants to see candidate again).

Total: /20

CIRCUIT C, STATION 4

Intraoperative complication – debriefing a patient

Candidate's instructions

The patient you are about to see is Kirsty Hadfield, aged 28 years, who was admitted as an emergency yesterday with a history of 6 weeks' bleeding following a normal delivery. Her haemoglobin was 9.8 g%. An ultrasound scan was performed which suggested the presence of an echogenic area in the uterine cavity. It was decided that she required an evacuation of the uterus.

She was taken to theatre by you for an evacuation of her uterus last night. Unfortunately, during this procedure the uterus was perforated and the bowel was pulled through the cervix. This was when you called the on-call consultant to theatre. You undertook a laparoscopy under supervision, which showed a perforation and bleeding, so you proceeded to a laparotomy. You oversewed the perforation, which was adjacent to a few small fibroids, and you wondered whether there could have been some degeneration of them to make the uterus so soft and consequently more susceptible to perforation. The rest of the pelvis looked normal. The sigmoid looked healthy and only required oversewing of the serosal surface.

You have 14 minutes to explain the findings to the patient and their implications for the future.

You will be awarded marks for:

- explaining the operative findings
- explaining future implications and management
- dealing with her concerns.

Role-player's brief

- You are Kirsty Hadfield, a 28-year-old woman who works as a legal secretary.
- Six weeks ago you delivered normally a live male baby at term, and have continued to bleed vaginally ever since. You have been fobbed off a few times by your GP with courses of antibiotics but have finally been admitted.
- You signed a consent form for evacuation of the uterus (D&C) but now have pain in your abdomen and have a pressure dressing over a wound. There is a drain and urinary catheter in place. You are concerned that they have taken away the uterus.

Prompts for questions

- 'What did you do, did you do a hysterectomy?'
- 'Why did this happen?'
- 'Why didn't you wake me up and discuss it?'
- 'What happens if I try for another baby?'
- 'Can I still breastfeed?'
- 'Did the fibroids have anything to do with it?'
- 'Why didn't you remove the fibroids?'
- 'Is this because people have fobbed me off with antibiotics?'
- 'I want to see the consultant' (become increasingly aggressive about having been operated on by a junior member of the staff and this happening)
- 'I want to complain.'

Examiner's instructions and mark sheet

Familiarize yourself with the candidate's instructions. The candidate is asked to:

- explain the operative findings
- discuss the implications and management for the future
- deal with the patient's concerns.

Score the candidate's performance on the mark sheet. The role-player will have a maximum of 2 marks to award the candidate. You should not interact with the candidate. Do not award half marks.

Explanation of the operative findings and procedures performed

- Reasons for the evacuation in the first place
- Concerns at the time of the evacuation
- The need for a laparoscopy once the bowel was pulled through the cervix
- The possibility of perforation of the uterus may be due to infection or degeneration of the fibroids
- Allow questions along the way
- Try to be open and non-defensive
- Bowel damage – the perforation was oversewn and should cause no problem
- Emphasize that the uterine cavity was empty at the end of the procedure

0   1   2   3   4   5   6

Discussion of implications and management

- Rest of pelvis was normal
- Short-term management
  - Allow to eat and drink
  - Drain and catheter out as quickly as possible
  - Mobilize and encourage early discharge
  - Short course of antibiotics
  - Venous thromboembolism (VTE) assessment
- Medium-term management
  - Wait until she has had a few normal periods before trying to get pregnant, though may want to wait longer in view of having a new baby
- Longer-term management
  - Would need to consider mode of delivery at 37 weeks
  - Most likely to go for a normal vaginal delivery
  - Discuss future types of contraception

0   1   2   3   4   5   6

Addressing patient concerns

- Management of the fibroids – risks of removing them at that time may have caused unnecessary bleeding
- Favour conservative approach unless become symptomatic
- Repeat an ultrasound scan in 3–4 months as the fibroids may have disappeared
- Answer questions about seeing consultant in the future
- Can continue breastfeeding (try to ensure timing to avoid maximum serum concentration)
- Patient Advice and Liaison Service (PALS) and complaints procedures

0   1   2   3   4   5   6

Role-player's score

0   1   2

(2 = role-player happy to see candidate again, 1 = prepared to see candidate again, 0 = never wants to see candidate again).

Total: /20

Postpartum haemorrhage – structured viva

Candidate's instructions

You are the registrar on duty and have just delivered Mrs Abbott by using a Kiwi cup. The delivery was reasonably straightforward, although you had to perform an episiotomy. You were concerned that there may have been some degree of shoulder dystocia, but using the McRoberts position, the baby was delivered without any delay. The third stage was straightforward. The episiotomy repair appeared straightforward.

Mrs Abbott is para 3, having had two full-term normal deliveries followed by an elective Caesarean section for an extended breech with failed external cephalic version. She was listed for a VBAC (vaginal birth after Caesarean section). She was admitted in spontaneous labour and progressed quickly in labour, but there were concerns about her CTG so you decided to expedite her delivery with the Kiwi.

You are called back to see Mrs Abbott 30 minutes later when the midwife finds her sitting in a pool of blood which she estimates is at least 500 mL. Her blood pressure (BP) is 90/60 mmHg and her pulse rate is 100/minute.

> **THIS IS A STRUCTURED VIVA. DURING A PERIOD OF 14 MINUTES THE EXAMINER WILL ASK YOU A SERIES OF FIVE QUESTIONS.**

Examiner's instructions and mark sheet

Familiarize yourself with the candidate's instructions and ask the questions as stated on this mark sheet. Do not prompt. Mark the candidates globally on each section, and do not give half marks.

1. What is your initial management of this patient?

- Call for help
- Rapid assessment of patient – vital signs (pulse/BP), palpation of the uterus
- Ensure intravenous access
- Emergency treatment of oxygen, plasma expanders
- Abdominal and vaginal examination (VE)
- Inspect the episiotomy if possible
- Control of bleeding (oxytocics, uterine massage)
- Ensure uterine contraction and assess effect on the volume of bleeding
- Urinary catheterization with hourly measurements of output
- Involve senior colleagues, anaesthetist and midwives

0   1   2   3   4

2. What investigations would you do?

- FBC
- Clotting screen
- Urea and electrolytes (U&Es)
- Cross-match 6 units of blood
- Check that the placenta has been checked to be complete

0   1   2   3   4

3. What is the diagnosis and, in this patient's case, what are the possible causes?

Provisional diagnosis is primary postpartum haemorrhage (PPH) due to:

- Atonic uterus
- Retained products or blood clot
- Unrecognized lower genital tract trauma
- Ruptured uterus from previous CS scar

0   1   2   3   4

4. You have massaged the uterus which seems to keep relaxing and so her bleeding persists. What do you do next?

- Needs examination under anaesthesia (EUA) to check cavity for retained products/clots
- Consent needed for EUA and possible hysterectomy
- Inform anaesthetist and theatre staff
- Ensure consultant is informed and ask to attend
- Ask anaesthetist if he would consider inserting a CVP (central venous pressure) line
- Systematic approach in theatre:
  - Ensure uterine cavity empty
  - Gently feel lower segment
  - Repair any previously undetected lacerations
- Use of oxytocics, ergometrine, hemabate as appropriate via PPH protocol
- May need Bakhri balloon insertion
- Keep estimates of input and output (blood loss and urine)
- Consider laparotomy if there is no improvement with the above measures:
  - repair rupture
  - vessel ligation
  - uterine brace suture (B Lynch type)
  - hysterectomy

0   1   2   3   4

5. What would your postoperative management involve if you need to do a laparotomy?

- May need transfer to intensive care unit (ICU)
- Antibiotics
- Transfusion as appropriate including FFP and cryoprecipitate depending on need
- Regular FBC/renal function and clotting
- Hourly urine output
- Thromboembolic deterrent (TED) stockings and reassess thromboembolic risk and manage accordingly
- Risk management form
- Debriefing of patient to explain what has been happening
- Follow-up to discuss this event and future pregnancies

0   1   2   3   4

Total: /20

Obstetric history with travel

Candidate's instructions

The patient you are about to see has been referred to your antenatal clinic by her GP. A copy of the referral letter is given below. Read this and obtain a relevant history from the patient, discuss the management of this pregnancy, and address any concerns she may have regarding it in 14 minutes.

The general examination of this patient is normal for her gestation.

Dear Doctor

Re: Tania Kaunas

Please see and book this 30-year-old Lithuanian woman for antenatal care. She has been in the UK for 3 years and speaks good English. However, she is a little vague about her obstetric history but appears to have one child and lost one child but we have no records. She is currently 20 weeks pregnant, which was confirmed by a first trimester ultrasound scan in your early pregnancy assessment unit and a recent detailed scan was normal.

Her history would appear to be otherwise unremarkable. She is keen to visit her grandmother in Lithuania for her 80th birthday and would like your advice.

Yours sincerely

Dr Lawrence

You will be awarded marks for:

- obtaining a relevant obstetric history
- establishing a plan of management for this pregnancy
- addressing any patient concerns.

Role-player's brief

- You are Tania Kaunas, a 30-year-old Lithuanian woman, who has been in this country for 3 years. You have been married for 7 years and work as a part-time learning support worker. You had trained as a teacher in Lithuania.
- Your periods are regular, bleeding for 4–5 days every 28 days. You have never had a cervical smear test.
- You smoke 5–10 cigarettes per day and drink only occasionally.
- You have no medical history of note. You are unaware of your blood group. There is no family history of note.
- This is a planned pregnancy. You had some bleeding in early pregnancy for which you had an ultrasound scan so are sure of your dates. Otherwise, there have been no other problems so far in this pregnancy. You are still worried because of previous problems.
- When you were aged 25 years you had a baby girl at 37 weeks' gestation. The pregnancy had been normal but you remember having a lot of pain and bleeding prior to going into the hospital, and when you arrived you delivered very quickly. The baby was 2.8 kg and needed admission to the neonatal unit for 48 hours.
- Two years ago you had another planned pregnancy but did not receive very much in the way of antenatal care for a variety of reasons. You did not see a doctor until about 28 weeks when you noticed that the baby had not moved for about 12 hours. You went to the hospital and the baby was found to be dead on scan. A labour was induced and you delivered a stillborn male infant weighing 2.3 kg after 12 hours. There was no post-mortem. There was not much in the way of explanation at home.
- You are keen to visit your grandmother next month for her 80th birthday and you want to know what advice the doctor would give you regarding airline travel.

Examiner's instructions and mark sheet

Familiarize yourself with the candidate's instructions. The candidate is asked to:

- take a relevant history
- establish a plan of management for this pregnancy
- address the patient's concerns.

Score the candidate's performance on the mark sheet. The role-player will have a maximum of 2 marks to award the candidate. You should not interact with the candidate. Do not award half marks.

History-taking

- General obstetric history – a planned pregnancy with good support?
- Check last period and expected due date
- Obstetric history
- Medical and surgical history
- Smoking, alcohol and drug history
- Smear history – may need opportunistic smear

0   1   2   3   4   5

Obstetric history

- History of first pregnancy – suggestive of a placenta abruption
- Normal fetal weight in first pregnancy
- Acknowledges the intrauterine fetal demise (IUFD) and the baby is heavy for the gestational age
- Possibly hydropic or macrosomic baby or the dates were incorrect and may want to check
- Discuss possible causes of the previous IUFD

0   1   2   3

Management in this pregnancy

- Need to check blood group and antibody status
  - May need tertiary referral depending on the levels
- Gestational diabetes screen
- Looking for non-immune causes of hydrops
  - Infection, e.g. parvovirus
  - Cardiac lesion

0   1   2   3   4   5

Air travel during pregnancy

- Usually not a risk to a healthy pregnant woman
- International travel all right up to 32–35 weeks; advise patient to carry her own notes with the expected date of delivery (EDD) and appropriate insurance
- Aisle seat over a bulkhead provides most space and a seat over the wing in the midplane region will give the smoothest ride
- Advise to walk every 30 minutes and flex and extend ankles frequently
- Safety belt to be fastened at pelvic level
- Fluids to be taken liberally because of dehydrating effect of low humidity in the aircraft
- Support stockings may be of use
- Important to exclude any potential problems before giving any further advice about travelling

0   1   2   3   4   5

Role-player's score

0   1   2

(2 = role-player happy to see candidate again, 1 = prepared to see candidate again, 0 = never wants to see candidate again).

Total: /20

Secondary amenorrhoea – structured viva

Candidate's instructions

Ms Janet Lansbridge is 32 years old and has been referred with a history of secondary amenorrhoea by her GP. She started her periods at the age of 13 years. Her periods were regular until she became pregnant at the age of 26, when she had a full-term normal delivery of a live female infant. She is anxious about the absence of periods as she has a new partner and they have been trying for a pregnancy over the past year.

Her brother had been diagnosed at the same time as her delivery with Hodgkin's lymphoma and he subsequently died. When she was 28 years old she developed a 'funny' feeling in the chest and was fobbed off by her GP that she was anxious because her brother had died from Hodgkin's disease. After having consulted the GP for about 12 months with similar non-specific symptoms, she was sent for a chest X-ray to placate her. However, this showed extensive shadowing and she too was found to have Hodgkin's lymphoma. She underwent intensive treatment and was advised to have a mirena coil fitted to avoid the risk of pregnancy. She is now clear of disease.

Her mirena coil was removed 12 months ago and she has not seen a period since that time. She recently complained of some hot flushes and some increase in the frequency at which she opens her bowels. She also feels she is becoming more hirsute.

Her mother had a total abdominal hysterectomy and removal of her ovaries for severe endometriosis when she was 42 years old and then commenced hormone replacement therapy (HRT).

> **THIS IS A STRUCTURED VIVA. THE EXAMINER WILL ASK YOU A SERIES OF FIVE QUESTIONS ABOUT THIS CASE OVER A PERIOD OF 14 MINUTES.**

Examiner's instructions and mark sheet

Familiarize yourself with the candidate's instructions. You have a series of five questions to ask the candidate. Ask the questions as written on the script and do not prompt. Do not award half marks.

1. What is the differential diagnosis in this case?

- Most likely premature menopause
- May be due to her chemotherapy
- Need to check she isn't pregnant
- Could have polycystic ovary syndrome (PCOS)
- Need to exclude other endocrinological causes

0   1   2   3   4

2. What investigations would you recommend?

- Check her BMI
- Serum FSH/LH/SHBG/testosterone
- Serum oestradiol
- Prolactin
- Pregnancy test
- Thyroid function tests
- Ultrasound scan of pelvis
- Progesterone challenge test

0   1   2   3   4

3. Her FSH and luteinizing hormone (LH) are raised 45 u/L and 33 u/L, respectively, her thyroid function tests were normal, and the pregnancy test was negative. What is the likely diagnosis and what would you do now?

- Premature menopause
- Would want to repeat the FSH and LH levels after 2 months
- Need to mention the fact that there is a small risk of becoming pregnant so in usual circumstance would need to exclude pregnancy
- Progesterone challenge test, but just check for pregnancy initially

0   1   2   3   4

4. Her progesterone challenge test was negative and her FSH remains elevated. In light of the history given, how would you manage her continuing care?

- Implications around the premature menopause
  - May need HRT long term
  - May want to find complementary medicine
  - May need to change lifestyle, e.g. more exercise and modify her diet
- Implications for her fertility
  - One could give advice only if it is sought
  - May need assisted conception with ovum donation
  - Consider adoption
  - Could possibly ovulate occasionally

0   1   2   3   4

5. What long-term consequences may she experience as a result of a premature menopause?

- Inability to conceive without reproductive technology
- Menopausal symptoms
- Osteoporosis – consult with the appropriate rheumatologists about bone densitometry in 2–3 years' time
- May have problems with bladder function
- Sexual function may be uncomfortable due to vaginal dryness
- Will have some cardiovascular implications

0   1   2   3   4

Total: /20

CIRCUIT C, STATION 8

Twin pregnancy – structured viva

Candidate's instructions

This is a four-part station and it follows the course of a twin pregnancy. At each stage you will be asked a question about the scenario.

Once you have dealt with each part of the question you should progress to the next part. You cannot go back to the previous section once finished. You have a total of 14 minutes to cover the four sections.

Marks will be awarded for answering the examiner's questions.

PART 1

Mrs JB, a 37-year-old woman, presents to the hospital emergency department. She is in her second pregnancy, having had a normal vaginal delivery of a live male infant at term. That baby weighed 2.2 kg. This current pregnancy is with a new partner and she has recently had in-vitro fertilization (IVF). She is now 8 weeks pregnant and has been unwell with morning sickness, which was far worse than in her first pregnancy. However, her main problem has been bleeding and she is very scared because of all the efforts she has gone through to become pregnant.

> **OUTLINE YOUR PROJECTED MANAGEMENT OF THIS PATIENT.**

PART 2

The ultrasound scan showed a monochorionic diamniotic twin pregnancy. Both fetal hearts are present and her bleeding settles. Her hyperemesis symptoms remain troublesome but she has controlled the situation with antiemetics and antacids. She was keen to go home and there was no reason for her to stay.

> **WHAT PARTICULAR AREAS WOULD NEED TO BE COVERED AT A BOOKING VISIT?**

PART 3

Mrs JB has progressed normally throughout the pregnancy. She has remained well apart from some of the minor symptoms associated with a twin pregnancy. She stopped work and also stopped smoking soon after her booking visit. The detailed scans of her twins were normal when performed at 20 weeks, and the growth has been maintained until 32 weeks' gestation.

At this visit her BP has crept up to 140/90 mmHg (booking BP at 11 weeks was 120/70). She has been asymptomatic and is currently on her soluble aspirin. Growth of the twins has been satisfactory, athough they are both under the 50th centile.

As she has been at home for most of the pregnancy she has had time to 'surf the net' and consequently she wants to discuss the possibility of a home birth.

> **WHAT WOULD BE YOUR ONGOING MANAGEMENT FOR THIS PATIENT?**

PART 4

The pregnancy has continued to progress and any concerns about her BP have not materialized. The babies' growth pattern has been maintained but they continue to be on the small side. She presents at the labour ward at 36+ weeks' gestation with spontaneous rupture of membranes and irregular contractions. The CTGs are essentially normal.

> **HOW WOULD YOU MANAGE THIS LABOUR?**

* In the exam, the candidate would see only one part at a time before moving to the next one.

Examiner's instructions and mark sheet

Familiarize yourself with the candidate's instructions. Ask the questions as they appear on the script and do not prompt. The scoring should be awarded globally.

PART 1

Outline your management of Mrs JB

- Main issues that need to be recognized:
  - Hyperemesis
  - Bleeding – threatened miscarriage
  - Anxiety due to the background of IVF
- Need to exclude any other relevant history:
  - Any other symptoms
  - Cervical cytology – could the bleeding be local, should have been done before the IVF cycle
  - Drugs usage/smoker
  - Check she has been using progesterone supplements
  - Has she been commenced on soluble aspirin
  - Any relevant medical history
- Examination:
  - General physical examination including BP and pulse rate
  - Needs a VE at some stage to assess the cervix
- Investigations:
  - FBC/U&Es
  - Liver function tests (LFTs)
  - Check urine for ketonuria
  - Ultrasound to assess viability
- Treatment:
  - Standard protocol with fluids – normal saline/Hartmann's
  - Antiemetics/antacids as indicated
  - Continue with progesterone supplementation
  - Rest

0 1 2 3 4 5

PART 2

What particular areas would need to be covered at a booking visit?

- Booking visit done by the midwife before 12 weeks' gestation
- Recognize monochorionic twins have a higher morbidity than diamniotic twins
- Also recognize maternal age and increased risk of Down's syndrome
- Detail maternal issues:
  - Check general symptoms including nausea, constipation, varicose veins
  - Random blood sugar
  - FBC and early recourse to commencing oral iron
  - Advise about smoking if an issue in view of previous small baby
  - Soluble aspirin needs to be discussed in light of previous intrauterine growth restriction (IUGR)
  - Ensure she is using her progesterone supplementation
  - VTE risk assessment at booking
  - Regular BP/urine checks
- Detail fetal issues:
  - Nuchal scan at 11–13 weeks
  - 2-weekly growth scans from 18 weeks onwards
  - Risk of twin-to-twin transfusion – implications
  - Aim to continue pregnancy to 38 weeks if possible, depending on growth

0   1   2   3   4   5

PART 3

What is your ongoing management for this patient?

- The main issues:
  - Raised BP
  - Growth of twins
  - Home birth
- Check symptoms: headaches, flashing lights, blurred vision, swelling
- Raised BP – need to check urine:
  - FBC, U&Es, LFTs, urate as baselines
  - 24-hour urine if significant proteinuria
  - May need mid-stream urine (MSU)
- Regular monitoring of the mother's BP, may need to start on antihypertensives
- Continue on soluble aspirin but should stop after 34 weeks

- May need to consider steroids if delivery is looking imminent, in which case inform paediatricians
- Regular CTGs and observations
- Weekly Dopplers after discussion with fetal medicine department
- Discuss home birth – advise against it but listen to patient's concerns

0   1   2   3   4   5

PART 4

How would you manage this labour?

- Maternal monitoring on partogram
- One-to-one midwifery care
- Need to review VTE assessment
- IV access
- Pain relief; advise epidural
- Group & save, recent Hb if one not available
- Fetal monitoring throughout the labour of both twins
- Check presentation of the first twin
- Inform paediatricians now
- Aim for vaginal delivery provided the first twin is a cephalic presentation
- Describe what should be done once first twin is born:
  - IV syntocinon
  - Examine vagina for presenting part
  - Controlled artificial rupture of membranes (ARM) at the height of a contraction
- Delivery of second twin:
  - Options depending on whether cephalic or breech
- Active third stage

0   1   2   3   4   5

Total: /20

Molar pregnancy – counselling with result

Candidate's instructions

The patient you are about to see is Mrs Astride, who is 40 years old. She had an evacuation of the uterus for what was thought to be a missed miscarriage about 2 weeks ago. The histology report has come back showing a complete hydatidiform mole. She was under your consultant's care 3 years ago when she had a Caesarean section for IUGR and PET (pre-eclamptic toxaemia); a live male infant was delivered at term. She is very concerned about having another child to provide a sibling for her son.

She is unaware of the histology report. You have 14 minutes to break to her the news and its implications. You are asked to discuss her further management and address her concerns.

Marks will be awarded for:

- explaining the diagnosis
- explaining the implications and further management
- addressing the patient's concerns.

Role-player's brief

- You are a 40-year-old social worker called Mrs Brenda Astride. You have one child who was delivered by Caesarean section 3 years ago because of BP problems. He was a little on the small side and weighed 2.5 kg at term.
- You are anxious to provide a brother or sister for him and so further fertility is very important to you.
- You have no major illness and there is nothing in your history of note.
- Four weeks ago you had a miscarriage and had the womb emptied with you asleep. You had had a lot of morning sickness that prevented you going to work. You then started bleeding heavily when you reached 12 weeks' gestation. You were admitted as an emergency with vaginal bleeding and the ultrasound scan had not shown a baby in the womb.
- As you have been brought back to discuss the result you have an inkling that all was not quite right. The doctor will break the news to you.

Prompts for questions

- 'Why has this happened?'
- 'Is there anything that I did to cause this, or anything I could have done to prevent it?'
- 'Do I need any further treatment?'
- 'What are the chances of it happening again?'
- 'Is there any chance of a further pregnancy?'
- 'Would it be worth going for IVF?'

Examiner's instructions and mark sheet

Familiarize yourself with the candidate's instructions. The candidate is asked to:

- explain the diagnosis
- explain the implications and further management
- address the patient's concerns.

Score the candidate's performance on the mark sheet. The role-player will have a maximum of 2 marks to award the candidate. You should not interact with the candidate. Do not award half marks.

Diagnosis explanation

- Acknowledge pregnancy loss/bereavement aspect
- Check that her bleeding has settled
- The diagnosis explained in simple terms and that it produces excess human chorionic gonadotropin (HCG)
- This may have caused excessive vomiting (it is also a way of monitoring the pregnancy)
- The diagnosis of molar pregnancy explained correctly – 90 per cent have duplication of haploid sperm XX and remainder dispermic XY; female nuclear DNA is inactivated (avoiding medical jargon)

0   1   2   3   4   5   6

Implications and further management

- Importance of further follow-up
- Registration with trophoblastic service (in the UK, Charing Cross, Sheffield and Dundee)
- There is a set protocol that they follow which includes reviewing the histology
- Patient will need a chest X-ray
- Follow-up is by checking beta-HCG levels, usually urinary
- Repeat serum level today
- Most of this is done by sending specimen pots to the patient to return so doesn't need to go to the centre unless problems with the HCG levels
- If HCG level is back to normal quickly then follow-up for only 6 months
- If slow return to normal then follow-up may be for 2 years – persistent trophoblastic disease in 10–15 per cent of cases
- 2–3 per cent may develop into choriocarcinoma but cure rate is high
- Advise against oral contraception as can affect the HCG assay

0   1   2   3   4   5   6

Candidate addresses concerns

- Emphasizes that it is not her fault and a fundamental problem with fertilization of the egg
- 80–85 per cent have a subsequent normal pregnancy
- 2 per cent risk of second molar pregnancy of whom 20 per cent risk have a third mole
- At the age of 40 years, no reason why she should need IVF if she has conceived normally on two previous occasions
- Risk of pregnancy loss increases with age, and increased risk of Down's syndrome
- Should not need any further treatment unless still bleeding, in which case may be worth repeating the evacuation of the uterus, or if the HCG is slow to return to normal

0   1   2   3   4   5   6

Role-player's score

0   1   2

(2 = role-player happy to see candidate again, 1 = prepared to see candidate again, 0 = never wants to see candidate again).

Results interpretation – preparatory station

Candidate's instructions

This is a preparatory station. You have a total of 15 minutes to read through the brief synopses of each case together with any associated investigation results. You will then meet the examiner and have 14 minutes to discuss all the cases.

For each case you will need to discuss:

- what further information you would need from the patient
- how you would explain the results to her
- an appropriate management plan for each case.

CASE 1

Ms Clements is 39 years old. She has been referred to your gynaecology outpatient clinic with a history of irregular bleeding over the previous 4 months. She has been taking oral contraception over the past 12 months. She has had one full-term normal delivery. Her last cervical smear test was 2 years ago and was normal. She is a smoker.

Results

- Ultrasound scan:
  - Normal-sized anteverted uterus, endometrium 4 mm, and midline not seen
  - Three echogenic areas within the cavity – possible blood clot or possible polyp
  - Both ovaries multifollicular
  - Normal adnexae

CASE 2

Clare Meacock is 20 years old and in the second year of a 3-year degree course at university. She presents with a history of secondary amenorrhoea for 18 months. She is also concerned about hirsutism, particularly on her forearms. Her menarche was at 13 years of age and her periods have always been a little erratic. Her height is 1.67 m and her weight is 43.8 kg, giving a BMI of 16.3.

Results

- LH: 4.7 U/L
- FSH: 9.3 U/L
- Prolactin: 205 mU/L (83–527)
- Testosterone: 2.8 nmol/L (0.5–3.0)
- Cortisol: 424 nmol/L (171–800)
- SHBG: 25 nmol/L (38–103)
- Ultrasound scan
  - Normal-sized anteverted uterus, clear cavity
  - Left ovary 22 × 15 mm, right ovary 24 × 14 mm
  - Multiple tiny follicles consistent with PCOS
  - Free fluid in the POD

CASE 3

Mrs Hutchinson, aged 37 years, returns to your clinic for the results of her fertility investigations. She has a regular cycle and no significant history of note.

Results

- Hysterosalpingogram: normal spill of dye through both tubes
- Day 21 serum progesterone: 72 nmol/L
- Sperm count:
  - Volume 1.5 mL
  - Count 8×10^6/mL
  - Motility 40 per cent
  - Progressive motility 50 per cent
  - Abnormal forms within normal limits

CASE 4

Mrs Jones, aged 59 years, was admitted last night with a history of postmenopausal bleeding (PMB) and discharge which has been happening over the past 3 years. She was unable to pass urine and has recently had difficulty in doing so. She has recently had an abnormal smear and is awaiting a colposcopy appointment. She has no other health problems or any relevant history. Her BP is 150/80 mmHg. Abdominal examination was unremarkable but vaginal examination revealed a frozen pelvis, with a friable mass on the cervix.

Results

- Hb: 8.3 g%
- WCC: 19.0×10^9/L
- Platelets: 641×10^9/L
- Na: 126 mmol/L
- K: 6.0 mmol/L
- Urea: 38.1 mmol/L
- Creatinine: 820 mmol/L

CASE 5

Mrs Naila Bibi, aged 41 years, recently underwent a hysteroscopy for heavy vaginal bleeding. She had recently been admitted with the bleeding and a haemoglobin of 6 g/dL. She is a non-insulin dependent diabetic on metformin. She has had three full-term normal deliveries in the past.

Results

- Histology: simple hyperplasia of the endometrium

CASE 6

Mrs Maria Bradbury is a 44-year-old woman with a 9-month history of amenorrhoea. She has had one early miscarriage and two full-term normal deliveries. Her current BMI is 25. She is not currently using any contraception.

Results

- Serum oestradiol: <20 pmol/L
- FSH: 69.4 U/L
- Prolactin: 238 mU/L

CASE 7

Abigail Heathcote is a 40-year-old woman who presented with a 5-year history of painful periods but the cycle is regular: 7 days' loss every 28 days. Over the past 3 months she has had some intermenstrual bleeding. She has had two full-term normal deliveries. On examination, the uterus is slightly enlarged to approximately 10 weeks' size.

Results

- Hb: 8.7 g%
- MCV: 63 fL
- Ultrasound scan:
  - Uterus anteverted and slightly enlarged
  - Endometrial thickness 10 mm
  - No other obvious abnormality detected
  - Ovaries look normal

CASE 8

Mrs Bridget Wright, aged 76 years, presents to the fast-track clinic. She has had some lower abdominal pain for which her GP arranged a scan. She has been reasonably fit in the past but has recently been diagnosed with atrial fibrillation and is taking warfarin. She has not had any abdominal surgery in the past.

Results

- Ultrasound scan revealed a 4 cm simple cyst on the right ovary; the other ovary could not be visualized in view of bowel gas. Small uterus with an endometrial thickness of 3 mm.
- Ca125 = 8

Examiner's instructions and mark sheet

Familiarize yourself with the candidate's instructions and the case summaries.

The candidates are asked to discuss with you:

- what further information he/she would want to know from the patient
- how he/she would explain the results to her
- an appropriate management plan for each case.

Each case is to be marked out of 5, so the final mark needs to be divided by 2 (rounding up) to give a score out of 20.

CASE 1

Questions

- What type of oral contraception – OCP or POP (progesterone-only pill)
- Any gastrointestinal upset that may affect absorption of the oral contraception
- Any other medication which may interfere with absorption
- What is her BMI

Explanation

Looks like endometrial polyps.

Options

- Hysteroscopy/D&C and polypectomy
- Location either outpatient or day case, depending on the patient
- Would mirena IUCD be a better option in view of her being a smoker?
- Has she had a pregnancy test?

0   1   2   3   4   5

CASE 2

Questions

- Why is her BMI so low?
- Does she have anorexia or an eating disorder?
- What are the patient's expectations?
- Does she need contraception?
- What are her stress levels at university?

Explanation

Most likely diagnosis is PCOS, but her low BMI may be a contributing factor. BMI <18 will usually cause the patient to be amenorrhoeic.

Options

- Depends on expectations of the patient
- OCP (Dianette) – clomid may be inappropriate at this time
- Consider inducing a withdrawal bleed with provera as it has been 18 months since last period, but exclude pregnancy initially
- Cosmesis for hairiness – e.g. waxing, electrolysis
- Warn of need for contraception
- Does the BMI need investigation – either malabsorption or psychiatric referral?

0   1   2   3   4   5

CASE 3

Questions

- Check the last menstrual period (LMP) as always a chance of pregnancy
- About the semen sample collection and any delay in getting it to the lab
- Partner's habits re. smoking and marijuana
- Type of job, undergarments, baths, illnesses

Explanation

- Patient's results normal
- Sperm count low, may reflect his health 2 months earlier
- Concern as to whether this is the highest or lowest count

Options

- Repeat sperm count at least once
- Possible need for andrology referral
- Decide what the couple want and discuss accordingly
- Intrauterine insemination (IUI) husband or donor, IVF/ICSI (intracytoplasmic sperm injection), adoption
- Depends on the couple's views but need to take age into account

0   1   2   3   4   5

CASE 4

Questions

- What was the smear abnormality?
- Does she have any pain?
- When did she last pass urine?

Explanation

Her anaemia is probably secondary to her PMB. She has renal failure, which needs to be treated.

Options

- Needs ultrasound scan to see if she has hydronephrosis
- Needs dialysis followed by insertion of nephrostomy tubes
- Referral to the urologists – need to establish a diagnosis and may need EUA, cystoscopy and sigmoidoscopy
- Will need imaging CT/MRI, biopsy and MDT review for ongoing management
- Most likely to be carcinoma of cervix and then will need chemo-radiotherapy

0   1   2   3   4   5

CASE 5

Questions

- When was her LMP?
- What is happening to the bleeding at present?
- What is her BMI?
- What are her thoughts about fertility?

Explanation

There is a premalignant lesion of the endometrium, but the risk of progressing is very low (approx. 1 per cent).

Options

- Options will depend on her fertility situation
- Medical treatment with mirena IUS (intrauterine system) and/or oral progestogens

- Would need repeat hysteroscopy and endometrial biopsy after 3 months of treatment
- Surgical option of hysterectomy, route depending on the clinical findings

0   1   2   3   4   5

CASE 6

Questions

- Hot flushes and night sweats
- Any other symptoms
- Has she seen any further bleeding
- Could she be pregnant and has a pregnancy test been done
- Any family history of early menopause and osteoporosis

Explanation

She is likely to be menopausal, but caution in view of age.

Options

- Repeat FSHs 3 months apart in view of age
- Treat symptomatically with HRT
- Would need contraceptive advice in view of age, depending on the repeat FSH level
- In the long term, she may need bone densitometry and appropriate management

0   1   2   3   4   5

CASE 7

Questions

- When was her LMP, does she pass any clots or experience flooding?
- What is her fertility expectation?
- What is her BMI, is it likely to affect the situation?
- Has she already had any treatment?
- In view of her anaemia, is she vegetarian and what is her diet like?

Explanation

The haemoglobin level is probably a reflection of chronic blood loss, likely to be menstrual but would need to consider other possible causes depending on symptoms.

Options

- Depends on her fertility status and what has been tried before
- Needs oral iron
- Hormonal or non-hormonal treatment, possibly mirena
- In view of anaemia, patient needs a hysteroscopy to exclude any endometrial hyperplasia and could assess suitability for mirena, ablation or possible vaginal hysterectomy

0   1   2   3   4   5

CASE 8

Questions

- Does she still have symptoms? If so, describe the nature and site of them
- What was the reason for the scan?
- Does she have any concerns?

Explanation

- She has been sent in as a target wait (2-week wait rule)
- The cyst looks benign and may not actually be causing her any symptoms
- RMI is very low but as target may consider an MRI

Options

- Will depend on patient and warfarinization
- Options include repeating scan in 3 months with a repeat Ca125
- Laparoscopic oophorectomy may be an option depending on symptoms, but warn that it may not resolve all her symptoms

0   1   2   3   4   5

Subtotal: /40
Divide score by 2:

Total: /20

Breaking bad news – Down's syndrome

Candidate's instructions

Ms Cropper has come to the antenatal clinic to discuss her Down's syndrome screening and chronic villus sampling (CVS) results. She had expected to see the consultant but he has been called away. You are left to counsel her and she has been waiting at least an hour already. At this station you are asked to counsel Ms Cropper and discuss the further management of this pregnancy.

Ms Cropper is 40 years old, in her first pregnancy, having tried for a pregnancy for the past 2 years. She is now at 14 weeks' gestation as it took her some time to come to terms with the nuchal result before deciding on having chorionic villus sampling.

The results of the quadruple test and the subsequent scan and chorionic villus sampling are as follows:

- nuchal thickness 4 mm at 11 weeks' gestation
- CVS result: abnormal – trisomy 21.

You will be awarded marks for:

- explaining the results from the CVS
- discussing the further management of this pregnancy
- providing appropriate counselling.

Role-player's brief

- You are Julie Cropper, a 40-year-old maths teacher in your first pregnancy.
- You had expected to see the consultant to discuss the chorionic villus sampling result, having had an increased nuchal thickness result on an early scan. You are disgruntled at the length of time you have waited and the apparently casual attitude of the staff you have come across to date. You eventually get to see the registrar (the candidate) who should introduce himself/herself. If not, ask the candidate exactly who he/she is and his/her level of experience.
- You are not convinced of the result as the couple who had the chorionic villus sampling before you looked 'far more likely to have a Down's syndrome baby than us' (your words). Could the results have been mixed up?
- The candidate should explore the results with you and the reason for having the screening in the first place (i.e. your age risk). All the results point to the diagnosis being correct.
- The options that you want to discuss are termination of pregnancy (TOP) and what it involves, and the possibility of continuing the pregnancy. The candidate should offer to arrange a paediatric consultation for you, but you should not lead the candidate in this particular area.
- You are upset and concerned about the possibility of future pregnancies and how, if you have a termination, you are going to cope with it mentally and how much time you will need off work.

Examiner's instructions and mark sheet

Familiarize yourself with the candidate's instructions. The candidate is asked to:

- explain the result from the CVS showing Down's syndrome
- Discuss the further management of this pregnancy
- provide appropriate counselling.

Score the candidate's performance on the mark sheet. The role-player will have a maximum of 2 marks to award the candidate. You should not interact with the candidate. Where the section is marked out of 4, then that section should be marked globally. Do not award half marks.

Discussion of results

- Apologize for the delay
- Explain the results and diagnosis, avoiding jargon
- Answer questions sensitively and without interrupting
- Explain the reason for the nuchal screening test in the first place (age-related)
- Explain that the diagnosis is compatible with life but the severity of the problem cannot be predicted
- Quality assurance is in place in the laboratory to ensure that the diagnosis is correct

0   1   2   3   4

Further management

- Discuss that the options are of termination or continuing pregnancy
- Offer paediatric consultation if that would help to make the decision
- National Down Syndrome Society may also be helpful
- As she is currently at 14 weeks' gestation, she does have time to think about the situation
- As it is not life-threatening, most would offer termination up to 20 weeks according to the abortion law (most obstetricians would advise making a decision before 20 weeks)

0   1   2   3   4

Continuing the pregnancy

- Routine care as for any normal pregnancy
- Would need a detailed scan at 20 weeks to exclude any possible structural anatomical defects that may affect her decision

- Routine antenatal care that would best suit her
- Attendant risks of being a primip and 40 years old

0   1   2   3   4

Decision on termination

- Explain that termination can be done up to 20 weeks' gestation
- Vacuum termination is probably inappropriate after 14 weeks
- Would need to sign a consent form before embarking on the process
- Would need to induce a mini-labour:
  - Mefipristone initially
  - Cervagem
  - Extra-amniotic termination if difficulty getting delivery with cervagem
  - Warn that it may take some time to happen
  - Warn that there is a risk of needing to have an evacuation of the uterus
  - Offer photos, hand and foot prints
  - Post-mortem if there have been any structural anomalies

0   1   2   3   4

Appropriate counselling

- Give option to come back after a time to think it over
- Counselling after TOP and offer appropriate bereavement counselling
- Follow-up and advice about trying to conceive another pregnancy

0   1   2

Role-player's score

0   1   2

(2 = role-player happy to see candidate again, 1 = prepared to see candidate again, 0 = never wants to see candidate again).

Total: /20

Pregnancy case – structured viva

Candidate's instructions

This is a four-part station, following the course of a woman's pregnancy. At each stage you will be asked a question about the scenario. Once you have dealt with each stage you should progress to the next. You cannot go back to a section once finished. You have 14 minutes to cover the four stages.

You will be awarded marks for answering the examiner's questions.

PART 1

Mrs HA is a 34-year-old Asian woman who has limited English. She is para 2+2.

Twelve years ago she had a Caesarean section (CS) in Bangladesh, the reason being unclear. That baby weighed 3.2 kg. Then she had a miscarriage prior to a further pregnancy 7 years ago. She had a spontaneous normal delivery, having had problems with gestational diabetes. That baby weighed 2.5 kg. Four years ago she had a pregnancy terminated at 10 weeks' gestation.

In her current pregnancy she was booked by a midwife at 10+5 weeks' gestation. Her body mass index (BMI) was recorded as 28, blood pressure (BP) 100/55 mmHg, haemoglobin 11.1 g%, mean corpuscular volume (MCV) 78 fL with normal electrophoresis. She had no other problems.

> **WHAT WOULD BE YOUR PLAN OF MANAGEMENT FOR THIS PATIENT?**

PART 2

Mrs HA is seen at 22 weeks' gestation, when her detailed ultrasound scan of the baby is normal. The pregnancy appears to be progressing well. However, she appears to have persistent 1+ proteinuria. Her glucose tolerance test (GTT) revealed a fasting blood sugar of 4.9 mmol/L, at 2 hours it was 9.6 mmol/L.

HOW WOULD YOUR PLAN OF MANAGEMENT CHANGE AT THIS STAGE?

PART 3

Mrs HA attends at 37 weeks' gestation. She has remained on a diet regimen to control her gestational diabetes, and her blood sugars appear to be reasonably well controlled with occasional high levels. She had attended for ultrasound assessment of the baby but failed to attend the antenatal clinic.

The scans performed at 28, 32 and 36 weeks showed normal growth, and at 36 weeks the estimated fetal weight was 3.1 kg. At this stage her haemoglobin was 10.1 g% with an MCV of 63 fL. The fetal presentation was cephalic.

WHAT WOULD BE YOUR PLAN FOR THE ONGOING MANAGEMENT OF THIS PATIENT?

PART 4

Mrs HA attends the labour ward at 38 weeks' gestation with a history of irregular contractions. She is unsure of whether her membranes have ruptured. BP is 140/90 mmHg. The presentation is cephalic with an engaged head, and on vaginal examination (VE) the cervix is 4–5 cm dilated with intact membranes.

WHAT IS YOUR PLAN FOR MANAGING HER AT THIS STAGE?

---

* Each stage would be seen after completing the previous one.

Examiner's instructions and mark sheet

Familiarize yourself with the candidate's instructions. Ask the questions as they appear on the script and do not prompt. The scoring should be awarded globally.

PART 1

What would be your plan of management for this patient?

- Mother:
  - GTT needs to be undertaken
  - Check the rest of her booking bloods, checking hepatitis/HIV and rubella status
  - Needs thromboembolic assessment
  - Vaginal birth after Caesarean section (VBAC) clinic attendance may not be necessary
- Fetus:
  - Down's screening with a nuchal scan
  - Will need a detailed scan at 20–22 weeks
  - Serial scans in the third trimester as she had IUGR in the second pregnancy despite the gestational diabetes mellitus (GDM)

0   1   2   3   4   5

PART 2

How would your plan of management change at this stage?

- GDM on the GTT: refer her to the diabetic team, probably best treated with diet alone but if it worsens then she may need to commence insulin
- Ensure ultrasound scans are booked for every 4 weeks
- Check her Hb at 28 weeks
- Persistent proteinuria requires mid-stream urine (MSU) plus a 24-hour urine for protein quantitation
- May require renal ultrasound depending on how the situation unfolds
- Aim to assess at 36 weeks for mode of delivery in view of previous CS
- Aim to deliver at 38–40 weeks' gestation depending on diabetic control and growth of the baby

0   1   2   3   4   5

PART 3

What would be your plan for the ongoing management of this patient?

- Mother:
  - Variable compliance and may need community midwife to visit
  - Need to emphasize the importance of good control of her blood sugars
  - Commence oral iron
  - Needs to decide on either an elective lower-segment Caesarean section (LSCS) or induction of labour (if the latter, then an induction date should be given)
- Fetus:
  - Growth has been good despite poor compliance
  - Important to stress to the woman that monitoring in labour would be needed

0   1   2   3   4   5

PART 4

What is your plan for managing her at this stage?

- Mother:
  - Plan to ensure she makes progress in the labour
  - Aim for a vaginal delivery provided she makes good progress and there are no fetal heart problems
  - Commence sliding scale of insulin along the lines of the department protocol
  - Recognize that the BP is significantly raised from the booking BP, so monitor
  - May want to check pre-eclamptic toxaemia (PET) bloods as a baseline
  - Routine urine testing for ketones and proteinuria
  - Analgesia
  - Artificial rupture of membranes (ARM)
  - Commence intravenous line/fluids
- Fetus:
  - Continuous monitoring
  - Fetal scalp electrode would need to be applied if problems

0   1   2   3   4   5

Total: /20

Antepartum haemorrhage – structured viva

This is a three-part station following the course of a woman who presents at 38 weeks' gestation with an antepartum haemorrhage. At each stage you will be asked a question about the scenario. Once you have dealt with each stage you should progress to the next. You cannot go back to a section once finished. You have 14 minutes to cover the three stages.

> **YOU WILL BE AWARDED MARKS FOR ANSWERING THE EXAMINER'S QUESTIONS.**

PART 1

You are the duty obstetric registrar on the labour ward. You have been asked to see Jennifer Eccles who has just been admitted with an antepartum haemorrhage. She had soaked her bed this morning and when she woke up was lying in a pool of blood and was very frightened. She has been 'blue-lighted' in by ambulance. It is estimated that she may have lost about 400–500 mL.

Mrs Eccles is 34 years old, in her second pregnancy, having had a full-term normal delivery of a live male infant weighing 3.4 kg. She is now 35 weeks' pregnant. She has been a compliant patient and attended all her antenatal classes. Her blood group is AB rhesus negative.

> **WHAT IS THE DIFFERENTIAL DIAGNOSIS IN THIS CASE? OUTLINE YOUR INITIAL MANAGEMENT OF THIS PATIENT.**

PART 2

On admission the patient's BP was recorded at 120/70 mmHg with a pulse rate of 100/minute. She was alert but appeared shivery and obviously anxious. She was distressed by the bleeding which appeared to be continuing. The pain appeared to be getting worse.

On abdominal examination, her uterus is tense and tender. It is proving difficult to hear the baby's heart beat with the Doppler ultrasound scan. However, you managed to see the heart beating with the ultrasound scan at approximately 110/minute.

> **HOW WOULD YOU MANAGE THE PATIENT AT THIS TIME?**

PART 3

VE reveals a 4 cm dilated cervix. You repeat the examination in theatre but the baby is not deliverable vaginally. Consequently, you perform an emergency CS with the patient asleep. A live male infant is delivered but is fairly floppy with Apgar score of 4 at 1 minute but 9 at 5 minutes. The cord pH was 7.1, the baby weighed 2.8 kg. The paediatricians decide to take the baby to the neonatal unit.

At the time of the CS there was a large retroplacental clot, and by the end of the procedure you estimate a total blood loss of 2.5 L. The anaesthetist has managed to keep on top of the fluids whilst the patient was asleep.

At the end of the procedure there is good haemostasis and you decide against insertion of a drain.

> **OUTLINE YOUR CONTINUED MANAGEMENT OF THIS PATIENT UP TO DISCHARGE.**

* Candidates would see only one section at a time.

Examiner's instructions and mark sheet

Familiarize yourself with the candidate's instructions and ask the questions as written. Please ask the questions as written and avoid prompting. Do not award half marks.

PART 1

1. What is the differential diagnosis in this case?

- Placental abruption
- Placenta praevia
- Vasa praevia (though unlikely if there is excessive bleeding as total fetal blood volume is unlikely to exceed 300 mL)
- Ruptured uterus
- Placental edge bleed
- Cervical tumour or other local causes

0   1   2   3

2. Outline your initial management of this patient

- A rapid assessment of the patient needs to be undertaken, checking her vital signs
- Is the bleeding continuing, and if so how much has been the overall volume loss
- IV access with 14-gauge cannulae
- Blood tests including full blood count (FBC), clotting, urea and electrolytes (U&Es), liver function tests (LFTs), cross-matching of blood (usually 4–6 units depending on the assessment)
- Once bloods taken, then give fluids i.v. (normal saline/Hartmann's) or Haemacel depending on the clinical picture
- Abdominal palpation for tenderness and auscultation for the presence of the fetal heart
- Review the notes to see if there are any underlying problems with the pregnancy
- Inform the labour ward consultant, anaesthetist and haematologist if it looks as though this is an abruption
- Further management depends on the clinical picture and the presence or absence of the fetal heart

0   1   2   3   4

PART 2

How would you manage the patient at this time?

- Diagnosis appears to be placental abruption
- Important to know what is happening with the fetal heart
- Cervical dilatation – needs a VE, either with speculum if there are concerns about the placental location or other local cervical causes, otherwise digital examination to see whether the cervix is dilating and vaginal delivery is a possibility
- If not, then – with a baseline bradycardia and the overall picture – needs a Code 1 emergency CS to deliver the baby before the fetal heart is lost
- Continue resuscitation on the way to theatre
- Need to restore circulating volume
- Consent form needs to be signed
- As well as personnel already mentioned, need to inform paediatrician and blood transfusion service as may need blood transfusion
- Risk of developing disseminated intravascular coagulation (DIC)
- Ensure someone is keeping the documentation going, especially with regard to input and output of fluids
- Will need catheterization, with hourly urine volume
- May need a CVP depending on the clinical situation
- If she develops a coagulopathy then that needs correcting in liaison with the haematologist
- As a rule of thumb, 4 units of blood to every 2 units of fresh frozen plasma (FFP) to every 1 unit of cryoprecipitate
- May need platelet concentrate if count <50, and cryo if fibrinogen <1.0 g/dL

| 0 | 1 | 2 | 3 | 4 | 5 | 6 | 7 | 8 |

PART 3

Outline your continued management of this patient up to discharge

Immediate

- Consider high-dependency treatment, but joint decision with the anaesthetist
- Continue monitoring of vital signs
- Continue intravenous syntocinon infusion over the next 6–12 hours, depending on the clinical picture

- Check all her blood tests (FBC, clotting, U&Es) as indicated or recommended by the haematologist
- Monitor urine output hourly
- Thromboprophylaxis assessment (anti-embolism stockings ± heparin)
- Mother will need anti-D, ask haematologists to advise about dose
- Risk management form as massive bleed

Prior to discharge

- Debrief patient about the events around the emergency delivery
- Advise about risks in further pregnancy

0   1   2   3   4   5

Total: /20

Clinical governance – preparatory station

Candidate's instructions

The following obstetric case resulted in the death of a baby. You have 15 minutes to read through the case report. You will then meet the examiner.

CASE STUDY

JT was a 23-year-old woman who booked at 16+ weeks' gestation at this hospital to have her first baby. This was her first pregnancy and it was planned. Her booking BMI was 42, placing her in a high-risk category for this pregnancy. She was too late for a nuchal scan. In view of her BMI, an appointment was made by the midwife to see the consultant anaesthetist. This appointment was made for 19 weeks' gestation but she failed to attend and the next available appointment was after she would have been expected to have delivered the baby. A GTT at this stage was normal.

JT did not appear to have any antenatal problems apart from an episode of reduced fetal movements at 33 weeks, but that seemed to resolve spontaneously. She was seen regularly throughout the pregnancy, alternating the visits between the midwife and the hospital antenatal clinic. All her observations were normal. In view of her body size a growth scan was arranged at 34 weeks' gestation which showed a normally grown fetus, with a cephalic presentation.

She self-referred to the Day Assessment Unit with further reduced fetal movements at term. A cardiotocograph (CTG) was undertaken and this was interpreted as 'suspicious'. Consequently, she was transferred to the labour ward. Her trace improved and it was decided that the labour should be induced.

She was reviewed by the obstetric consultant on the labour ward. A 30-minute CTG was performed and it appeared to improve. It was decided to induce the labour at this time on the labour ward. The cervix was closed but 50 per cent effaced; 2 mg Prostin was inserted into the vagina.

One hour later, at 8.30 pm, the CTG became suspicious with a complicated tachycardia. At this stage the cervix was 2 3 cm dilated, and an emergency CS was recommended as it would probably take 5–6 hours for the cervix to become fully dilated. However, at this stage, neither JT nor her mother were agreeable to a CS at that time. The possible adverse outcome for the baby was explained. An hour later, the CTG had become pathological and the patient continued to decline a CS.

At 10.00 pm, JT finally agreed to a CS. Unfortunately at this time, another patient was having an emergency CS. The obstetric consultant discussed with the labour ward coordinator the possibility of opening the second theatre but it was felt that there were not enough midwifery staff to support this action. The obstetric consultant decided to stay behind to perform the section even though no longer on call. The consultant informed the anaesthetist on duty (ST2) who did not see her (JT) immediately as he was busy in theatre. He eventually saw her at 11.00 pm. On assessment, the anaesthetist identified some potential problems for intubation of the patient and so he made the decision to provide a spinal anaesthetic.

JT was transferred to theatre on a bed at 11.15 pm, and the spinal was commenced at 11.45 pm after the anaesthetist tried unsuccessfully to insert a second intravenous line. He then took about 40 minutes attempting to perform the spinal anaesthetic in different intervertebral spaces and using a variety of positions before calling for help from the ITU registrar.

The ITU anaesthetist was an ST3 and he arrived at 12.30 am and asked the labour ward anaesthetist to contact the consultant on call in view of the complications due to JT's obesity. The consultant on call advised a general anaesthetic (GA) but the second registrar managed to site the spinal at the last attempt at 12.45 am.

JT had a sudden hypotensive episode and required the administration of ephedrine. The CS was commenced at 1.00 am.

There had been consistent difficulty in monitoring the fetal heart due to JT's size, and this was further hampered by the positioning of her during the spinal procedure. The midwife had listened to the heart rate intermittently and at the start of the section it was recorded as 156/minute.

The baby was delivered at 1.05 am with no signs of life. Resuscitation was attempted by the paediatric team, but was discontinued at 1.35 am after the consultant paediatrician had discussed the situation with the parents. The cord blood gas results indicated chronic hypoxia.

On reflection, it appears that more importance was given to the possible complications from the CS and the anaesthetic for the mother due to her obesity than to the clinical consequences of the delay in delivery of the baby.

YOU WILL MEET THE EXAMINER TO ANSWER FOUR QUESTIONS:
- What were the main factors affecting the outcome in this case?
- What other factors contributed to the adverse outcome in this case?
- What areas of notable/good practice can you identify?
- What recommendations would you make on reviewing this case?

Examiner's instructions and mark sheet

Familiarize yourself with the candidate's instructions and ask the questions as written on the script. This station is about clinical governance and reflecting on an adverse obstetric event. Do not prompt the candidate. Do not award half marks.

What were the main factors affecting the outcome in this case?

- Delay in the patient being reviewed by the anaesthetist
- Delay in taking the patient to theatre once the patient had consented
- Delay in theatre due to the anaesthetic registrar's lack of experience with an obese patient
- Delay in seeking help from another anaesthetist

0   1   2   3   4

What other factors contributed to the adverse outcome in this case?

- Patient not seen antenatally by an obstetric anaesthetist (she was referred as per the protocol but cancelled her appointment)
- Patient and family's decision to decline a CS initially
- Patient's high BMI complicated the administration of an anaesthetic
- Patient's BMI and position adopted for the spinal procedure prevented the fetal heart being monitored continually
- Concerns were more around the mother than the fetus

0   1   2   3   4   5   6

What areas of notable/good practice can you identify?

- Community midwife at booking did an appropriate antenatal risk assessment and referred the patient appropriately
- Comprehensive obstetric and midwifery care was provided antenatally
- Consultant obstetrician recognized the need for senior medical attendance and so stayed on duty to deliver the patient
- Consultant paediatrician was present for the attempted resuscitation

0   1   2   3   4

What recommendations would you make on reviewing this case?

- An agreed guideline to open a second theatre on the labour ward at any time when it is indicated
- Important to escalate concerns to a higher level
- Multidisciplinary guideline for the care of obese women during their pregnancy and during their labour – should adopt the CMACE/RCOG Obesity Guideline
- Look at an increase in antenatal obstetrics anaesthetist services
- Review anaesthetic cover on the labour ward

0   1   2   3   4   5   6

Total: /20

Fertility issues

Candidate's instructions

The patient you are about to see was referred to your outpatient clinic by her GP. A copy of the referral letter is given below. You have 14 minutes to read the letter and obtain a relevant history from the patient. You should discuss an appropriate management plan and answer the patient's concerns.

The Surgery
Longdale Lane
Lindby Dale

Dear Doctor

Re: Geraldine Shepherd, aged 43 years

Thank you for seeing this patient, who is now 43 years old and has recently remarried. She came to see me requesting to see a gynaecologist concerning her fertility as she is worried that 'her biological clock is ticking along at the rate of knots'. She is relatively new to our practice but in view of her age does not want to wait unnecessarily.

Many thanks

Dr Stainsby

You will be awarded marks for:

- obtaining a relevant history from the patient
- discussing an appropriate management plan
- addressing the patient's concerns.

Role-player's brief

- You are Geraldine Shepherd, a 43-year-old architect, who has recently been married to Don, a history teacher, who has just reached the big five-zero!
- You want to have a baby together, but all has not been plain sailing as you have recently been treated for a chlamydial infection at the local department of sexual health. They performed a cervical smear test which was negative.
- Your periods are regular, lasting 4 days with a 30-day cycle. You have had one child in the past who is 18 years old. You cannot remember whether there were any problems. You had a full-term normal delivery and the baby weighed 3.4 kg. Don has two grown-up children.
- You are both busy people and tend to have intercourse mainly at the weekends and when on holiday.
- You have a glass of wine most nights with your evening meal unless you are working late, plus an occasional cigarette but nothing regularly. Neither of you uses any recreational drugs.
- You do not have any history of medical or surgical problems. If you are asked any other questions not covered in this briefing, then the answer should be that it is either normal or not relevant.

Concerns

The candidates have been instructed to deal with your concerns. You should ask the following questions when asked about those concerns:

- What are my risks if I do become pregnant?
- What are the risks for the baby now I am 43 years old?
- What would you recommend if and when I do become pregnant?

Examiner's instructions and mark sheet

Familiarize yourself with the candidate's instructions. The candidate is asked to:

- take a relevant obstetric history
- discuss an appropriate management plan
- address the patient's concerns.

Score the candidate's performance on the mark sheet. The role player will have a maximum of 2 marks to award the candidate. You should not interact with the candidate. Do not award half marks.

Relevant history

- Age of patient and partner
- LMP and cycle length
- Obstetric history
- Does the partner have any children
- Frequency and timing of intercourse
- Any sexually transmitted diseases (STDs)
- Previous abdominal surgery (appendix, CS)
- Any medical problems – BP or diabetic problems in previous pregnancies
- Last cervical smear
- Medication and allergies
- Social – smoker, alcohol and recreational drugs of both her and partner

0   1   2   3   4   5   6

Plan of management

- Check ovulation – mid-luteal progesterone
- Day 2 FSH – ovulatory reserve
- Tubal patency – hysterosalpingogram (HSG)
- Partner's sperm count
- May consider screening for rubella/hepatitis/HIV and STD screen in view of recent chlamydial infection
- Advise on coital frequency and timing
- Folic acid

0   1   2   3   4   5   6

Address patient concerns

- Maternal risks
  - Reduced fertility
  - Risk of tubal damage due to the Chlamydia
  - Increased risk of ectopic pregnancy
  - Thromboembolic risk increased and may need to make alterations to her lifestyle
  - Increased risks of gestational hypertension, gestational diabetes, antepartum haemorrhage
- Fetal risks
  - Increased risks of miscarriage
  - Increased risk of Down's/Edwards/Patau's syndromes as age increases
  - If partner >50 years, then increased risk of Apert's syndrome
- Antenatal care
  - Advise early ultrasound scan for location and viability
  - CVS
  - Fetal anomaly scan
  - Tailor the care to the patient
  - GTT at some stage
  - Thromboembolic risk assessment at booking
  - May decide to avoid post dates

0   1   2   3   4   5   6

Role-player's score

0   1   2

(2 = role player happy to see candidate again, 1 = prepared to see candidate again, 0 = never wants to see candidate again).

Total: /20

Management of ectopic pregnancy – structured viva

Candidate's instructions

You are the SpR on call for gynaecology. A 25-year-old woman has presented with a history of 6–7 weeks of amenorrhoea, vague pain in the right iliac fossa and some vaginal bleeding. Her periods are usually regular but she cannot quite remember when the last one occurred as she and her partner were trying for a pregnancy and she had assumed that they had been successful.

Her pregnancy test is positive and an ultrasound scan was performed. The findings show a live ectopic pregnancy in the right fallopian tube, with some fluid in the Pouch of Douglas (POD).

The examiner will ask you four questions on the management of this patient. You have 14 minutes in which to answer them.

Examiner's instructions and mark sheet

Familiarize yourself with the candidate's instructions. You have four questions to ask the candidate as they are written. Do not prompt.

What features in this patient's case would suggest that she should be dealt with surgically?

- The stability of the patient's condition
- The live ectopic in the tube
- Fluid (potentially blood) in the POD
- Impression that it is not a case for medical management

0   1   2   3

You decide she needs to go to theatre, so what key areas would you want to check before that happens?

- Intravenous access is in place
- FBC and group & save have been organized
- Ensure there are no problems with blood transfusion if needed
- Check that the consent has been signed and that the patient understands what procedure is likely to be undertaken
- Explain risks of the procedure
- Explain that this is a potentially life-threatening condition
- Any history of previous pelvic surgery

0   1   2   3   4

Describe your surgical approach

- Positioning of the patient in Lloyd Davies stirrups and urinary catheter inserted
- Prepare the skin with an appropriate antiseptic solution, and drape the patient
- Testing of the equipment
- Insertion of the Veress needle and the laparoscope
- Where the other ports will be sited and how they are inserted
- Initial assessment of the pelvis and abdominal cavity
- Photographs recommended
- Operative technique used and the reasons behind using that particular method
- Check haemostasis

- Consider washout, anti-adhesion measures and the possible use of a drain, depending on the findings
- Comprehensive operation notes

0   1   2   3   4   5   6   7

How would you manage the patient postoperatively?

- Review the patient and explain the procedure once the patient is able to understand
- At patient debriefing, show the photographs from the procedure
- Check FBC
- Check beta-hCG levels have gone back to normal
- Discuss the bereavement reaction
- Discuss future fertility and the risk of another ectopic pregnancy (1 in 8)
- Discuss the type of suture and the need for them to be removed if causing troublesome symptoms

0   1   2   3   4   5   6

Total: /20

Secondary amenorrhoea – role play

Candidate's instructions

You are about to see Jane McKenstrie who has been referred by her GP with a history of secondary amenorrhoea. She has had two hormonal profiles performed about 6 weeks apart, and both series showed significantly elevated FSH and LH levels with very low oestradiol levels. The results suggest the possibility of premature ovarian failure.

You have 14 minutes during which you need to:

- take a relevant history
- explain the possible diagnosis and its implications
- discuss an appropriate management plan.

Role-player's brief

- You are Jane McKenstrie, a 25-year-old history PhD student who has not had a normal menstrual period for 18 months. You weren't particularly worried about this, as you are keen on exercise and are quite slim. You are aware that low BMI can be related to absent periods. You have also been under stress as you are writing up your thesis.
- You started your periods at the age of 14 years and they were regular until you were 21 years old when you graduated with your bachelor's degree. At that time you took up exercise and started with rowing as you are keen to row in the Olympics. For the following 2 years your periods were irregular and your last normal period was about 18 months ago.
- You haven't noticed any other symptoms but went to see your GP 8 weeks ago about this problem and you had some hormonal blood tests taken. These blood tests have been repeated with no change in their values. You have been referred by your GP to discuss the implications of the situation.
- You are currently writing up your PhD in history. You are well and have been in hospital previously on only one occasion when you had your appendix removed at the age of 6 years. You have never been pregnant.
- You are currently sexually active and you have been with your partner over the past 2 years. You are using condoms for contraception and have noticed some vaginal dryness with intercourse recently.
- You do not take any medication, and have no allergies. You had a cervical smear test taken when you were 25 years old. Your mother stopped her periods at the age of 38 and you are an only child. Your grandmother had a deep vein thrombosis (DVT) and pulmonary embolus at the age of 42.

Concerns

- You want a diagnosis.
- You are very concerned about your fertility.

Examiner's instructions and mark sheet

Familiarize yourself with the candidate's instructions. You have no involvement in this station except for marking the candidate. Allow the role-player to give a mark out of 2 at the end of the station. Do not award half marks.

Taking a relevant history

- Age
- Menstrual history including menarche
- Obstetric history
- Current medication
- Weight loss and BMI
- Family history
- Current occupation
- Exercise levels
- Cervical smear test
- Fertility issues
- Other medical problems
- Smoking and alcohol history

0   1   2   3   4   5   6

Explaining the possible diagnosis

- FSH levels significantly raised suggests premature ovarian failure
- Short-term/immediate risks are around menopausal symptoms of vaginal dryness, hot flushes
- Intermediate problems are related to fertility and how that may affect her relationship with her boyfriend
- May need to consider ovum donation/surrogacy/adoption
- Long-term problems will relate to osteoporosis and increased risk of cardiovascular disease

0   1   2   3   4   5   6

Discussion of an appropriate management plan

- Investigations:
  - Repeat the FSH, check prolactin and thyroid function tests
  - Check FBC and U&Es to exclude any potential renal problem
  - Auto-antibody screen
  - Check chromosomes – possible Turner's mosaic

- Transvaginal ultrasound scan looking for any ovarian activity
- Baseline bone densitometry at some stage
- Treatment options:
  - Consider hormone replacement therapy (HRT) or combined oral contraceptive pill
  - Lifestyle changes including diet.

0   1   2   3   4   5   6

Role-player score

0   1   2

(2 = role-player happy to see candidate again, 1 = prepared to see candidate again, 0 = never wants to see candidate again).

TOTAL: **/20**

Postoperative pelvic abscess – role play

Candidate's instructions

You are about to see a 26-year-old secretary, Michelle Graham, who had a CS 8 weeks ago. She had her CS for fetal distress and was discharged home on day 4 despite her temperature being slightly raised. She continued to feel unwell with lower abdominal pain as well as feeling hot and cold. Three weeks after her CS she went to see her GP.

At that time she was very tender in the left iliac fossa and was transferred to hospital for further management. Investigations revealed that she has a large pelvic abscess in the left iliac fossa and a retained swab was seen on abdominal X-ray in the same area. She underwent a laparotomy and was discharged from hospital a week later. She has been given an early appointment to discuss her case. The obstetrician who performed her original CS is on vacation and you are the only person available to see her.

You have reviewed her notes. This was her second pregnancy and it appeared uneventful antenatally. She had had a previous full-term normal delivery with her first pregnancy. That baby weighed 3.4 kg. This time she went into spontaneous labour at 39 weeks' gestation, but at 6 cm dilatation the fetus developed late decelerations on the CTG. A fetal blood sample was taken and the pH came back as 7.19. She therefore had an emergency CS with delivery of a live male infant in good condition who weighed 4.3 kg. There was a lot of bleeding at the left uterine angle which required extra suturing. The swab count at the end of the procedure appeared normal.

You have 14 minutes during which you should:

- answer her questions
- deal with her concerns.

Role player's brief

- You are Michelle Graham and work as a secretary.
- You have just had your second baby delivered by CS, which was not straightforward. You are annoyed and upset that a swab was left inside your abdomen at the time of your section and you know that this is not acceptable practice. You have come to the clinic today expecting to see the obstetrician who did your section but found that she is on vacation.
- You found the delivery extremely traumatic as you had been concerned about the baby's heart rate. You had seen the rate dipping on the monitor. The section was performed with great haste under a spinal anaesthetic and you were aware that there were problems with bleeding at the time. You could overhear the conversations of the doctor doing the procedure.
- Following the delivery, you were slow to recover. You were upset that you were sent home on day 4 as you really didn't feel up to it. Nobody seemed to take any notice of you on the ward despite having a temperature when you were discharged.
- When you got home, you continued to feel unwell and experienced a lot of pain on your left side. You had episodes of feeling hot and then cold, especially during the night.
- When you went to see your GP, he acted very quickly and you were readmitted to hospital and required a further operation. Basically, you feel that your care was negligent. You found that nobody really explained what had happened particularly well. You have come today for an explanation and have a series of questions that you want answered.
  - Was the person who did the operation competent to be doing a CS on her own?
  - How do you explain that the swab count appeared correct but one was left in my abdomen?
  - Why was I discharged early despite feeling unwell and having a temperature?
  - Will this affect my future fertility if I want more children?
  - I plan to take this further and will be registering a complaint and seeking legal advice. Who do I contact?

Examiner's instructions and mark sheet

Familiarize yourself with the candidate's instructions. You have no involvement in this station except for marking the candidate. Allow the role-player to give a mark out of 2 at the end of the station. Do not award half marks.

'Was the person who did the operation competent to be doing a CS on her own?'

- Deal with the situation empathically
- Explain that the specialist registrars (SpRs) are all competent and are all assessed on their competencies before undertaking Caesarean sections alone
- There is always a designated labour ward consultant on duty
- Usually if there are technical difficulties then the SpR or the coordinating midwife will call for senior help
- Apologize that the surgeon involved is not available

0   1   2   3   4

'How do you explain that the swab count appeared correct but one was left in my abdomen?'

- Explain the WHO process of checking the patient into theatre and at the end of the surgery
- Acknowledge that the swab was left inside
- Swab count appeared correct at the end of the procedure
- Acknowledge a mistake has been made and a full investigation will take place, but that will be at a higher level
- Her baby was big and there may have been an extension of the incision on the uterus which caused the bleeding and made repair and haemostasis difficult

0   1   2   3   4

'Why was I discharged early despite feeling unwell and having a temperature?'

- Usual policy is to discharge women after 3 days
- It may have been considered that she would sleep and recover better in her home surroundings
- Early discharge may have been thought appropriate to avoid hospital-acquired infections

0   1   2   3

'Will this affect my future fertility if I want more children?'

- It is difficult to say for certain at this stage
- Ask how she would like to pursue this issue
- Options include considering HSG at 6 months or so post surgery
- Consider diagnostic laparoscopy and dye at some point in the future
- Patient tries for another pregnancy and do investigations if unable to fall pregnant within a specified length of time
- Explain that if she does become pregnant she may be at risk of an ectopic pregnancy, and so an early ultrasound scan would be indicated

0   1   2   3   4

'I plan to take this further and will be registering a complaint and seeking legal advice. Who do I contact?'

- Advise of complaints procedure and involvement of PALS (Patient Advice and Liaison Service)
- A full investigation will have been commenced in view of the case triggering a risk management alert
- Offer to provide name and address of chief executive
- Avoid being defensive
- She might be best advised to register the complaint first and then seek legal advice (once the legal team are involved then disclosure of the investigation may be delayed)

0   1   2   3

Role-player's score

0   1   2

(2 = role-player happy to see candidate again, 1 = prepared to see candidate again, 0 = never wants to see candidate again).

Total: /20

Polycystic ovary syndrome – structured viva

Candidate's instructions

> **THIS IS A STRUCTURED VIVA ABOUT PCOS.**

You have seen a 28-year-old nulliparous woman in the gynaecology clinic and have just presented her case to your consultant. You think she is likely to have polycystic ovary syndrome (PCOS), though she has had no investigations to date as she failed to attend for an ultrasound scan appointment and only had her blood tests performed today when she arrived at the hospital.

Your consultant (the examiner) will ask you a series of eight questions about the condition of PCOS. You have 14 minutes during which the examiner will ask you these questions.

Examiner's instructions and mark sheet

Familiarize yourself with the candidate's instructions. You have eight questions to ask the candidate. Read the questions exactly as they are written on the mark sheet. Avoid prompting the candidate. Do not award half marks.

1. What symptoms do women with polycystic ovaries usually exhibit?

- Infrequent periods – oligomenorrhoea
- Infertility
- Hyperandrogenism
- Hirsutism
- Acne
- Obesity

0   1   2   3

2. How do you diagnose PCOS?

- Exclude thyroid dysfunction, congenital adrenal hyperplasia, hyperprolactinaemia, adrenal tumours and Cushing's syndrome
- Rotterdam criteria: two of the three parameters which include:
  - Ultrasound showing either 12 or more peripheral follicles or increased ovarian volume >10 cm^3
  - Oligo- or anovulation
  - Clinical or biochemical signs of hyperandrogenism

0   1   2   3   4

3. What baseline tests will you request for your patient?

- Thyroid function tests
- Serum prolactin
- Free androgen index (total testosterone divided by sex-hormone-binding globulin (SHBG) times 100 to give a calculated free testosterone level)
- If total testosterone >5 nmol/L, then 17-hydroxyprogesterone should be measured and androgen-secreting tumours excluded
- If there are suspicions of Cushing's then this should be investigated according to local protocols

0   1   2   3

4. What do you think are the important aspects of PCOS that you need to discuss with the woman at this stage?

- She should be informed of the long-term risks of developing type 2 diabetes
- Sleep apnoea risk increased if BMI raised
- Increased risk of cardiovascular disease

0   1   2

5. What are the implications of PCOS if she decides she wants a pregnancy?

- She should be screened for gestational diabetes <20 weeks' gestation and managed accordingly
- Other problems related to raised BMI (e.g. hypertension/operative delivery)

0   1   2

6. If she does have PCOS, what risks might she have for cancer in the future?

- Increased risk of endometrial hyperplasia and carcinoma
- Regular withdrawal bleeds are recommended

0   1   2

7. What strategies would you recommend to the patient for the reduction of long-term consequences of PCOS?

- Advise exercise and weight control
- Insulin-sensitizing agents (e.g. metformin) may be useful
- Weight-reduction drugs may be helpful in reducing insulin resistance

0   1   2

8. Is there any place for surgery in patients with PCOS?

- Ovarian drilling should be reserved for selected infertile women with an ordinary BMI
- Bariatric surgery may be a possible option depending on local protocols

0   1   2

Total: /20

Audit – preparatory station

Candidate's instructions

The clinical lead for gynaecology has noted an increased number of wound infections in patients who have had an abdominal hysterectomy. The nursing staff have looked at some of the cases and noticed that they have not all been given antibiotics at the time of induction of their GA.

You are asked to design an audit, for which you have 15 minutes.

Examiner's instructions and mark sheet

Familiarize yourself with the candidate's instructions and the headings below. The candidate has 14 minutes to discuss his or her audit plan with you. Avoid prompting, and do not award half marks.

Defining the audit topic

- The use of intravenous antibiotics on induction of GA in women undergoing abdominal hysterectomy

0   1

Preaudit preparation

- Identify resources and convene a multidisciplinary group
- Contact the clinical risk and audit service
- Systematic review of evidence: literature – e.g. Medline, Cochrane, National Clinical Guidelines, Microbiology input
- Register the audit project

0   1   2   3

Define a standard

- Define the proportion of compliance that constitutes good practice (100 per cent) – i.e. all patients should be given intravenous antibiotics at induction of GA for their abdominal hysterectomy
- May need to define which antibiotic regimen should be used depending on microbiology advice

0   1   2

Data collection

- Decide whether to do a retrospective or prospective audit (a small retrospective audit may be useful in this situation to explore any possible difficulties)
- Define target of either time or number of cases to be of value
- Define the audit sample (all patients undergoing the operation)
- Consider any other reasons for wound infection, BMI, co-morbidities including diabetes, indication for the procedure, length of surgery
- Design a proforma to collect valid and reliable data
- Pilot the proforma

- Collect data
- Ensure data entered onto a spreadsheet
- Appropriate analysis and interpretation

0   1   2   3   4   5   6

Implement changes to improve care

- Feedback to individuals and units involved in the care of these patients
- Identify areas that need change (e.g. individuals, organizational changes, preoperative changes to optimize patient prior to surgery, change antibiotic regimen)
- Identify sources of resistance to change and anticipate potential problems – proactive approach
- Review medical practice as discussed above and use appropriate forums for that process
- Disseminate changes and new standards via email, newsletters, noticeboard bulletin, flyers, grand round-type meeting
- Define a time period for the implementation of these changes

0   1   2   3   4   5   6

Reaudit

- Define a suitable timeline for re-audit, usually within 12 months of changes
- Re-audit results would need to be re-evaluated to see if further changes are necessary to further improve clinical outcome

0   1   2

Total: /20

INDEX

abdominal pain, premature labour 107–10
abnormal smear 135–8, 207
Abortion Act (1991) 35, 165
adenocarcinoma, endometrial 59–63
air travel when pregnant 185–9
alpha-fetoprotein (AFP) 33, 34
amenorrhoea 207
   secondary 191–3, 206, 245–8
anaemia 163, 166, 207, 208, 211, 212–13
anencephaly 33–8
antepartum haemorrhage 223–7
antibiotics at GA induction 257–9
Apert's syndrome 239
aspirin 196, 198
audit 48–51, 257–9
autonomy 166

bereavement 89–91
bleeding
   intermenstrual 97–9, 207–8, 212–13
   irregular while on oral contraceptive 205, 209
   postmenopausal 119, 129, 206
   see also haemorrhage
blood pressure control 146–52
blood transfusion 226
   Jehovah's Witnesses 155, 166

BMI, low 206, 209–10
breaking bad news 33–8, 59–63, 215–18
breech delivery 157–60

Ca125 level 171, 174, 175
Caesarean section 131–3
   elective for placenta praevia 19–22
   emergency 224, 230, 249, 251
   review after 16
cancer
   cervix 137, 207, 211
   counselling 59–63
   endometrial 59–63
capacity 163, 166
carbamazepine 98, 99
cardiotocograph (CTG) 229–30
   not reassuring/abnormal 139–44
   premature pregnancy 72
case notes 39–46
cervical carcinoma 137, 207, 211
cervical ectropion 124, 129
cervical polyps 124, 129
cervical smear, abnormal 135–8, 207
chlamydial infection 237, 238, 239
choriocarcinoma 203
chorionic villus sampling 215, 217
clinical governance xviii, 229–33

clinical management skills xvii
    early pregnancy problem-
        management 9–12
    ectopic pregnancy 241–3
    gynaecology problem 73–6
    obstetric history and management
        69–72
clinical skills xvi
colposcopy counselling 137
communication skills xvii
    ectopic mismanagement 23–6
complaints 252
confidentiality 165
contraception
    emergency 93–6
    epilepsy medication 98, 99
    under-16s 162, 165
cord pH 169
corpus luteal cyst 9, 12
counselling skills xvii
    bereavement 89–91
    cancer 59–63
    colposcopy 137
    molar pregnancy 201–4
    prenatal 77–80
    termination of pregnancy for
        Down's syndrome 218
cystic fibrosis testing 77–80

Data Protection Act (1998) 165
death of baby 229–33
debriefing patient on intraoperative
    complication 177–80
delivery suite prioritization 13–18
delivery unit board 14, 101
dementia 163, 166
diabetes, gestational 219–22
discharge policy 251

Down's syndrome 198, 204, 215–18,
    239
dysfunctional uterine bleeding (DUB)
    121, 129
dyskaryosis 118, 129, 135

early discharge 251
early pregnancy problem-
    management 9–12
ectopic pregnancy
    explain laparoscopy 153–6
    management 241–3
    mismanagement 23–6
    pelvic abscess 252
Edwards syndrome 239
emergencies
    Caesarean section 224, 230, 249,
        251
    shoulder dystocia 167–70
    uterine inversion 81–3
emergency contraception 93–6
endometrial adenocarcinoma 59–63
endometrial hyperplasia 207, 211–12
endometrial polyps 205, 209
endometriosis 40, 125, 129
epilepsy medication, OCP use 98,
    99
ethical issues 161–6
evacuation of uterus 177–80
external cephalic version,
        contraindications 160

fertility issues 235–9, 252 see also
    infertility
fetal death 89–91
fetal distress 143
fibroids 2, 66, 68, 73–6, 163, 177, 180

flying when pregnant 185–9
follicle-stimulating hormone levels
    127, 129, 192, 245, 247
Fraser guidelines 165
free androgen index 254

genetic testing for cystic fibrosis
    77–80
gestational diabetes 219–22
Gillick competency 165
good practice xvi
GP letters, prioritization 117–30
grand multip, viva 145–52
gynaecological history 1–7
gynaecology management problem
    73–6

haemorrhage
   antepartum 223–7
   postpartum 181–3
HELPERR 169–70
hirsutism 191, 206, 210
history-taking
   comprehensive history taking
      xv–xvi
   gynaecological history 1–7
   obstetric history xv–xvi, 52–8,
      69–72, 185–9
Hodgkin's lymphoma 191
human chorionic gonadotropin
    (HCG) 203
hydatidiform mole 201
hydrostatic method 82
hysterectomy
   antibiotics at GA induction
      257–9
   subtotal 76
   total abdominal 66–7, 76, 163
hysterosalpinogram 42

hysteroscopy 75, 76

in-vitro fertilization (IVF) 26, 44,
    195
induced labour 229–30
infertility 39–46, 120, 129, 206, 210
interactive viva 145–52 *see also*
    structured viva
intermenstrual bleeding 97–9, 207–8,
    212–13
intraoperative complications, patient
    debriefing 177–80
intravenous antibiotics at GA
    induction 257–9

Jehovah's Witnesses 153, 155, 163,
    166

labour
   induction 229–30
   obese mother 229–33
   premature 16, 107–10
   twin pregnancy 199
labour ward prioritization 100–5
laparoscopy 67, 153–6
legal issues 161–6, 252
LETZ 138
levonelle 95
logical thought xvii
loop excision of the transformation
    zone 138
low BMI 206, 209–210
low sperm count 42, 45, 46, 206, 210
luteinizing hormone levels 127, 129,
    192, 245

malposition/malpresentation 16
management *see* clinical management
    skills

marking scheme xviii
Mauriceau Smellie Veit manoeuvre
160
McRobert's position 169
meconium liquor 14, 16
medication history xvi
menopause 207, 212
premature 191–3
Mental Capacity Act (2005) 166
Mirena IUCD 209, 211
miscarriage 9–12
molar pregnancy 201–4
MRCOG Part 2 examination,
structure xiv
myomectomy 76

neonatal death 229–33

obesity 121, 129, 229–33
objective structured clinical
examination see OSCE
obstetric emergencies
Caesarean section 224, 230, 249,
251
shoulder dystocia 167–70
uterine inversion 81–3
obstetric history-taking xv–xvi, 52–8,
69–72, 185–9
operating list prioritization 84–8
oral contraceptive pill
epilepsy medication 98, 99
irregular bleeding 205, 209
prescribing to under-16s 162, 165
OSCE (objective structured clinical
examination)
marking scheme xviii
structure xiv–xviii
osteoporosis 193
O'Sullivan's method 82

ovarian cyst 171–5, 208, 213
ovarian drilling 255

Patau's syndrome 239
pelvic abscess 249–52
pelvic floor exercises 115
pelvic mass 122, 129
pelvic pain 125, 129
perforated uterus 177–80
periods, painful and heavy 2, 73, 163,
166
placenta praevia 19–22
placental abruption 226
polycystic ovary syndrome 206,
209–10, 253–5
postmenopausal bleeding 119, 129,
206
postoperative pelvic abscess 249–
52
postpartum haemorrhage 181–3
Potter's syndrome 162
Pouch of Douglas 153, 171, 241,
242
pregnancy
air travel 185–9
early pregnancy problem-
management 9–12
gestational diabetes 219–22
grand multip, interactive viva
145–52
molar pregnancy counselling
201–4
structured viva 219–22
twin pregnancy 195–9
premature labour 16, 107–10
premature menopause 191–3
premature ovarian failure 245–8
premature prelabour rupture of
membranes 69–72

premenstrual syndrome 27–31
primary postpartum haemorrhage
    181–3
prenatal counselling 77–80
preoperative ward round 65–8
pre-senile dementia 163, 166
prioritization xvii
    delivery suite 13–18
    GP letters 117–30
    labour ward 100–5
    operating list 84–8
progesterone challenge test
    192–3
prolactin 127, 129
prolapse 123, 129
provera, withdrawal bleed 210
pruritus vulvae 126, 129

renal failure 206–7, 211
results
    incorrect labelling 45
    interpretation 205–13
retained swabs 249, 251
reverse Woods screw manoeuvre
    170
Rhesus negative 55
role-playing stations xv, xvi, xvii,
    xviii
Rotterdam criteria 254
rubella immunization 55
Rubin manoeuvre 169

secondary amenorrhoea 191–3, 206,
    245–8
semen analysis 42
serum AFP 33, 34
sex worker 54
shoulder dystocia 167–70

smear test abnormality 135–8,
    207
sperm count 42, 45, 46, 206, 210
steroids 16, 110, 152, 199
stillbirth 89–91
structured viva xviii, 19–22, 181–3,
    191–3, 195–9, 219–22, 223–7,
    241–3, 253–5 see also interactive
    viva
subtotal hysterectomy 76
surgery
    Caesarean section 131–3
    debriefing patient on
        intraoperative complication
        177–80
    ectopic pregnancy management
        241–3
    elective Caesarean for placenta
        praevia 19–22
swab, retained 249, 251

tachycardia 143
teaching station 167–70
termination of pregnancy 35, 162,
    165–6, 217, 218
test results
    incorrect labelling 45
    interpretation 205–13
total abdominal hysterectomy 66–7,
    76, 163
twin pregnancy 195–9

ultrasound scan 9, 42, 205, 206, 208
    audit 48–51
urinary incontinence 111–15, 123,
    129
urodynamics 114
uterine inversion 81–3
uterine perforation 177–80

vasa praevia 225
viva, interactive 145–52 *see also* structured viva
vulval itching 126, 129

waiting list prioritization 84–8

ward work
   labour ward prioritization 100–5
   preoperative ward round 65–8
WHO checklist 22
withdrawal bleed 210
Woods screw manoeuvre 170

T - #0838 - 101024 - C288 - 234/156/13 - PB - 9781444121841 - Gloss Lamination